The

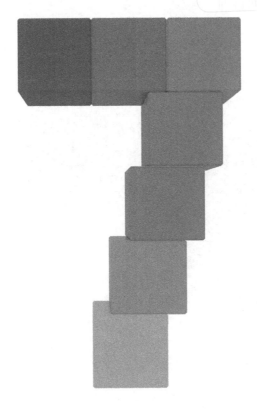

STAGES

of a

DENTAL PRACTICE LIFE CYCLE

The

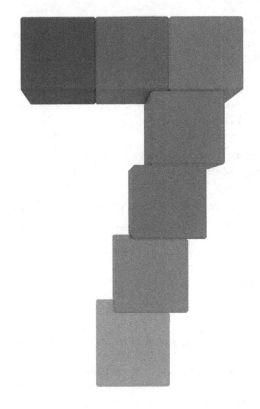

STAGES

of a

DENTAL PRACTICE LIFE CYCLE

MICHAEL A. PINCUS, D.D.S.

Advantage®

Published by Advantage, Charleston, South Carolina.
Member of Advantage Media Group.

ADVANTAGE is a registered trademark and the Advantage colophon is a trademark of Advantage Media Group, Inc.

Printed in the United States of America.

ISBN: 978-159932-370-1
LCCN: 2014933262

This publication is designed to provide accurate and authoritative information in regard to the subject matter covered. It is sold with the understanding that the publisher is not engaged in rendering legal, accounting, or other professional services. If legal advice or other expert assistance is required, the services of a competent professional person should be sought.

Advantage Media Group is proud to be a part of the Tree Neutral® program. Tree Neutral offsets the number of trees consumed in the production and printing of this book by taking proactive steps such as planting trees in direct proportion to the number of trees used to print books. To learn more about Tree Neutral, please visit **www.treeneutral.com**. To learn more about Advantage's commitment to being a responsible steward of the environment, please visit **www.advantagefamily.com/green**

Advantage Media Group is a publisher of business, self-improvement, and professional development books and online learning. We help entrepreneurs, business leaders, and professionals share their Stories, Passion, and Knowledge to help others Learn & Grow. Do you have a manuscript or book idea that you would like us to consider for publishing? Please visit **advantagefamily.com** or call **1.866.775.1696**.

I would like to thank my wife, Jeanette, and our two children, Scott and Erica, for giving me the motivation to go to work every day.

I would like to thank my father for teaching me to have integrity.

I would like to thank my mother for inspiring me to be a dentist.

I would like to dedicate this book to Dr. David Jackson—a great dentist, mentor, and friend. Dr. Jackson taught me how to run a dental practice and gave me the confidence to go out on my own.

TABLE OF CONTENTS

WHY I'M WRITING THIS BOOK

W e've modernized dental technology and medicine, but there's nothing modern about the practice of dentistry itself. The earliest evidence of dental treatment dates back to 7000 BC. Teeth with holes made by primitive dental drills were discovered in the skulls of people of the Indus Valley civilization, dating from 5500 to 7000 BC.

As the technology has continued to evolve, mankind has searched for ways to deliver less painful, effective, aesthetic and efficient dental treatment. In 500 BC Hippocrates and Aristotle wrote about tooth decay and gum disease, extractions, and the use of wires to stabilize loose teeth. Farmers and monks practiced dentistry in the Middle Ages. Claude Mouton first described a gold crown in 1746. In 1760 an English immigrant, John Baker, became the earliest medically trained dentist in America when he set up what is believed to have been the first dental practice in America, in the city of Boston.

Paul Revere placed the first dental advertisements in a Boston newspaper, offering his dental services. In 1844 Horace Wells discovered that nitrous oxide could be used for anesthesia. In 1859, 26 dentists in Niagara Falls formed the American Dental Association. William Redkin discovered the X-Ray in 1895. In 1957 John Morton developed the high-speed hand piece. Dental insurance came into being in the '50s. In the '90s, aesthetic dental treatment and lasers came to the forefront, further expanding the range of dental modalities available to the public.

All of these discoveries, as well as the ability to deliver multiple treatments in an increasingly competitive market, have placed a tremendous emphasis on the capacity of practitioners to deliver care efficiently. Helping you understand the different stages of a dental practice and the different strategies to manage each stage efficiently, effectively and professionally is the purpose of this book.

Dental practices, like all businesses, go through different phases, similar to phases of a person's life. The seven stages of a dental practice life cycle are:

SEED

START-UP

GROWTH

ESTABLISHED

EXPANSION

MATURE

EXIT

It is critical to learn what upcoming focuses, challenges and financial resources you will need to succeed. This book will be a reference and a guide through your practice's journey.

1

SEED

"Start where you are. Use what you have. Do what you can."

—ARTHUR ASHE

The seed stage of your practice life cycle is when your business is just a thought or an idea. This is the very conception of your dental career. This idea could have happened in high school, the second year of dental school, or any time you have considered starting your practice of dentistry.

CHALLENGE

Most dental practices will have to overcome the challenge of market acceptance and pursue one niche opportunity. Be careful not to spread financial resources too thin.

FOCUS

In the seed stage, the focus should be on matching practice opportunity with your skills, experience and passion. Other focal points include deciding on practice structure, finding professional advisors, and business planning.

FINANCIAL RESOURCES

Early in your dental career, after leaving the cocoon of dental school, you will have to make the transition from parents' support, student loans and part time jobs to life as a professional. Strategies will need to be developed to aid in that transition monetarily, socially and emotionally.

CHALLENGE OF MARKET ACCEPTANCE

Coming out of dental school is similar to when babies leave the nest to go into the wild. Although a new dentist is capable of performing good dental treatment, your skills are just evolving—and you must compete in a marketplace against excellent, experienced dentists who will call you a colleague but will consider you competition. How will you develop your niche? Why would patients flock to you? If you know the answer to these questions, you probably have the confidence to start a practice on your own. If you don't know the answers, it would be unwise to spend a fortune on an unrealistic dream.

These days, most young dentists don't open practices the way I did when I got started. They come out of school with such enormous debts that their options are limited, and the expense of opening a two-chair office today is about $400,000—even without buying the property.

When you start out, unless you have massive capital (or rich parents), it is a great idea to get your feet wet by working for someone else. You have a number of choices: You can be an associate in a private practice; you can be an associate in a large group corporate practice; you can join the military; or you can work in a private institution, one that might specialize in children, for instance. These are some examples of employment opportunities. I am sure there are more.

If you are dead set on owning your own practice, review this checklist before you decide on ownership as your career choice.

Are you confident in your ability to:

- ❑ perform simple extractions;

- ❑ perform simple molar endo in a timely manner;

- ❑ perform basic crown and bridge, with the understanding that continuing education is imperative for completing restoration, occlusion, and cosmetics as quickly as possible;

- ❑ understand that continuing education in implant restoration and implant placement brings skills and services that may not necessarily distinguish and separate you from your peers but may place you in a reasonably competitive position;

- ❑ manage a staff, schedules, human resources, and so on (have you ever balanced your checkbook?);

- ❑ take continuing education in orthodontics, botox treatment, snore appliances, laser treatments, anything that patients might be exposed to by the media if you really want to develop your niche quickly?

It also may not be a bad idea to take a personality profile at this stage of your thought process to help you better understand your needs, capabilities and desires. Meyers-Briggs or DISC are both good.

For more on DISC training, visit:

https://www.discprofile.com/what-is-disc/overview/

For more on Meyers-Briggs, visit:

www.myersbriggs.org

If you answered yes to all of these questions, skip to the part about buying your own practice.

If not, most young dentists accept positions as associates in

- private dental practices;

- corporate dental practices;

- military practices;

- institutions (public health, VA hospitals, pediatric clinics, dental schools).

A realistic month in the life of a dentist in the seed stage looks like this:

WEEK 1

MONDAY

Your lab partner in dental school reports to you that his real estate agent has located an ideal spot in the middle of town, two blocks from the dental school. He has contacted a dental supply house regarding equipment, and he is ready to sign the lease.

TUESDAY

You make a note to yourself to contact your uncle, who has a friend who knows a dentist, to talk about options after graduation.

WEDNESDAY

Written exams all day. You are close to getting paid to do dentistry, but you still have to concentrate on graduating first.

THURSDAY

Your friend in the next bay tells you he has accepted an associateship with a friend of the family back home.

FRIDAY

A recruiter from the military is at the dental school today to talk about the benefits of being a dentist and an officer in the military. You think it is interesting that you can take a military residency, gain some experience, and get paid—not bad.

WEEK 2

MONDAY

You wonder all weekend how your lab partner can afford to open an office. Doesn't he have student loans?

TUESDAY

Your fiancé tells you she really wants to move back to her hometown. You wonder if they need another dentist in her hometown.

WEDNESDAY

Your last bridge requirement doesn't seat and needs to be remade. Getting all of your requirements completed by graduation is going to be tight.

THURSDAY

As you struggle to finish your requirements, your lab partner tells you he has completed all of his and is going upstairs to do a sinus graft in the oral surgery graduate suite.

FRIDAY

A local dentist speaks today at the practice management class about options after dental school. Best info, most interesting class of the week. You feel you have a plan.

WEEK 3

MONDAY

Fully motivated, you fill out the application from the military regarding a career as a naval officer/dentist. You fill out requests from a large corporate dental chain that offers great benefits and guaranteed income. You respond to Craigslist for all want ads from dentists needing associates. You are going to show your lab partner.

TUESDAY

Your final requirement is a new denture patient who brings in a bag of five sets of dentures for you to replicate. Your prosthodontics professor, whom you don't like, is at the end of the bay, chuckling. So is your lab partner.

WEDNESDAY

Your mother calls to tell you she would be so happy if you practiced in her hometown. Unfortunately, your mother and fiancé don't live in the same hometown.

THURSDAY

While you are doing a wax try on your denture patient, your lab partner walks by and announces he is going upstairs to place six implants and an apicoectomy on number three. He giggles as he hears your patient say these teeth make her look like a rabbit.

FRIDAY

Meeting with financial affairs office to get info on student loan payoff options.

WEEK 4

MONDAY

Thank you, Lord. All cases are seating properly and denture wax-up is approved. There is an e-mail from your personal dentist back home. He heard you were graduating and he is considering an associate. Yippee! When you tell your lab partner, he tells you he can't decide whether to accept a teaching fellowship at Harvard, the ortho residency at Michigan, partnership with his uncle, or going out on his own. Your thoughts are: 1) Am I going to invite him to my graduation party? 2) Would strangulation be a reason to prevent you from graduating?

TUESDAY

Interview with corporate dental chain goes well. You are feeling better about getting a job after graduation and it feels good.

WEDNESDAY

Your bridge seats and your denture case is almost done. You have all of your board patients lined up. You speak to your personal dentist and make an appointment to meet. You know you would be a great fit in his practice. You wanted to become a dentist partly because of him.

THURSDAY

You get a copy of *Dental Economics* today and see the survey of average salaries of dentists by region. Your hometown is in the region with the highest income. You tell yourself you are not going to be average anyway.

FRIDAY

Happy Hour after school. Everyone is excited to talk about his/her plans after graduation.

FOCUS ON MATCHING CAREER OPPORTUNITIES WITH SKILLS, EXPERIENCE AND PASSION

Whether starting your own practice, or working for someone else, *it is important to establish a team of professional advisors*. You should have an accountant, lawyer, insurance advisor, and financial planner. The best way to start to build this team is to interview referrals from any of these professions. Once you find one you are comfortable with, ask that professional for the other referrals. Do not be afraid to ask up front what these professionals' fees are and how they calculate fees. Be prepared to pay for advice. Any free advice is usually not worth the price you paid for it.

Good financial, insurance, legal and accounting plans are imperative to build your path to success. A young dentist might ask why financial advice is necessary before any real income is earned. Think of it as a complex treatment plan of a full mouth rehabilitation case. You would never start without a treatment plan. Your team can also help with your decision of ownership versus associateship.

PRIVATE PRACTICE ASSOCIATESHIP

There are pros and cons to being an associate in a private practice. If you work for a private doctor, typically, you're going to be working for a dentist who might be in his forties or his fifties. It can be great experience, observing how to run a staff, interact with long time patients, and get real-time clinical training. A senior dentist could take a real interest in helping you develop your skills for the good of his practice and if he has a genuine interest in teaching a young colleague, this can be great. There is also a chance that he is going to want you to buy his practice down the line. If it is in an area where you can develop the existing practice and continue to develop your own niche in a still-growing area, this can also be great. If no growth is possible, you can spend a fortune on a depreciating asset. Not great. A senior dentist, who has devoted a lifetime to building a practice, will have a tremendous tendency to overvalue the practice. Be careful not to overpay for something that may have already peaked. View a dental practice like a stock. Buy low, sell high. A thriving practice looks great to a young associate, and very romantic to think about how great life will be when you are the senior doc, but it is much harder to maintain than it seems. Have your team evaluate any deal. It is okay to listen to your gut but go into a private practice relationship with eyes wide open.

CORPORATE PRACTICE

Joining a large corporate practice has become a much more viable option in the last few years for many reasons.

- Gaining clinical experience with less personal responsibility
- Stable salary
- Insurance and retirement benefits
- Possible financial support for continuing education
- Ability to pursue other opportunities without leaving behind a real personal attachment

The downside of corporate dentistry is:

- The impersonal nature of an ever-changing patient base;
- The corporation may think more of the bottom line than the dentist, often dictating laboratories to use, supplies and even the types of treatment to perform, taking the young doctor out of his comfort zone;
- Limited control of work schedule, assistants to pair with;
- Lack of personal identity (rather than being Dr. Jones, you are more like a mere employee at XYZ dental office).

MILITARY PRACTICE

The military can be a great option for a young dentist. The military often pays for dental education, offers retirement benefits, offers the prestige of being a military officer, has excellent health-care benefits for the dentist and his family, and often places the young dentist in a residency for great clinical experience.

MEDICAL INSTITUTIONS

Institutional settings, such as a children's clinic and the VA, are very similar to military employment and can offer similar benefits.

BUYING A PRACTICE

You have considered all options of associateship. You have reviewed my checklist regarding "readiness" to own a practice in a competitive environment. Your mind is made up. You are going out on your own! Now what? Do you start from scratch or buy an existing practice?

In 1982, when I started my practice, I had worked for a large clinic for about six weeks. I quickly decided this was not the environment for me and I quit (or was fired, I forget). I found a great job working as an associate in a private practice and worked there full-time and part-time as I built and established my practice.

I started my private practice with a friend from dental school. We each held our part-time jobs as we established our practice. In the early eighties, interest rates were sky high and it was not easy for us to get a loan, yet we had no fear about starting a practice from scratch. It seemed as if everyone was doing it and we never considered buying an existing practice. In today's environment, if you are going out on your own, I would strongly suggest buying an existing practice for the following reasons:

- More competitive environment today, making it more important to hit the ground running;

- Easier to get a loan; banks like to see existing cash flow;

- Inherit a staff that could help train a young dentist in office management. This is about a 50/50 proposition as a benefit, because sometimes the staff is the reason the office is being sold in the first place. So be ready with a rapid replacement plan;

- An existing office already has finished space, which is a large cost;

- May have an advantageous lease, or it may not, so be considerate of the lease;

- Takes the suspense and drama out of picking equipment, computers, office design, paint color, coffee pot, uniform colors, etc. These decisions can be overwhelming in addition to all the other decisions a young practitioner must make.

If you need more convincing that buying an existing practice is a better idea than starting from scratch, notice how the large corporations acquire practices more often than they start new ones. Corporations have investors and investors like to see cash flow. If it is good for them, it is good for you.

FINANCIAL RESOURCES

As you make the transition from dental student to professional, many changes are often happening in your personal as well as professional life. You may be getting married. If married, you may be starting a family. You probably have student loans. Your personal financial strategy should involve short-term and long-term goals. Short-term goals will include food, shelter, car payments, insurance … the day-to-day stuff. Long-term goals include student loan payoffs, saving for a house, new cars, even country club membership. Long-term goals need to wait a little. It generally takes two to four months to get your dental license to begin to practice. Resist the urge to run up your credit cards. Be patient and as frugal as possible. Part-time jobs and living at home with parents is common for a few months and may be a way to ask your parents or family for a loan against future earnings. They probably don't want you moving in with them as much as you don't want to move in with them. Be patient and do whatever it takes until you start practicing. Be confident in the fact that although it seems as if, since dental school, many of your friends have taken off and left you in the game of life, you soon will catch up and pass them.

This is a great career you are about to start! If you have decided on buying an existing practice, where do you find one? Dental brokers and dental journals are all over the Internet. Local supply houses are in the know and are a great source of referral, and often know of practices that are for sale. Brokers and suppliers are also good sources for referral for practice financing.

Be aggressive in telling people your intentions of buying a practice and opportunities will come looking for you. Decide on a location. First, decide where you want to live. The practice should be within a reasonable driving distance but not necessarily the neighborhood where you live. Look for opportunities for the growth of the practice. I love suburban and even rural areas. Swim in blue water (where other fish aren't swimming). Have your team evaluate the deal. Find agreeable financing and *jump*.

Follow this checklist prepared by my friend Dan Lewis, the best practice broker in America.

PURCHASER'S CHECKLIST

1. SECURING THE PRACTICE ACQUISITION LOAN

- ❏ Gather the necessary documentation:
    - ❏ Prepare a cover letter describing the opportunity;
    - ❏ personal financial statement;
    - ❏ personal living expenses budget;
    - ❏ tax returns of seller (three years);
    - ❏ tax returns of purchaser (three years);
    - ❏ cash flow projections for business;
    - ❏ current year income and expenses of practice;
    - ❏ practice appraisal.

- ❏ Obtain insurance coverage for loan securement:
    - ❏ life insurance in the amount of the loan;
    - ❏ use existing policy;
    - ❏ obtain new policy;
    - ❏ obtain insurance policy;
    - ❏ collateral assignment form;
    - ❏ personal disability policy;
    - ❏ monthly benefit to equal loan payment;
    - ❏ verify ability to substitute business overhead policy;
    - ❏ obtain contents insurance for purchased assets;

- ❑ obtain workmen's compensation policy (optional).

❑ Make application with third party payers:

- ❑ PPO providers (Delta, MetLife, etc.);

- ❑ capitation and Medicaid providers (approval may take 45–60 days).

2. RESOLVING PRACTICE PURCHASE CONTINGENCIES

❑ Meet with landlord to secure new lease or lease assignment:

- ❑ Have personal financial statement available.

- ❑ Get letter of financing approval.

❑ Meet with staff of seller in group and individual meetings:

- ❑ Emphasize your plan to retain employees without immediate changes.

- ❑ Obtain ideas for practice growth.

- ❑ Secure verbal commitments for retention of employees.

3. PREPARING TO ASSUME BUSINESS

❑ Interview and select accountant:

- ❑ Determine level of services needed.

- ❑ Have contract of purchase and sale reviewed.

- ❑ Review tax allocations of assets.

❑ Interview and select attorney:

- ❑ Determine level of services needed.

- ❏ Have sale documents reviewed.

- ❏ Have loan documents reviewed.

- ❏ Establish business form/documentation.

❏ Choose form of practice operation:

- ❏ sole proprietorship

- ❏ S corporation

- ❏ C corporation

- ❏ professional association (PA)

❏ Apply for tax ID # (employer identification number):

- ❏ Call (800) 829-4933, or

- ❏ Use Internet application at http://www.irs.gov.

❏ Interview and select bank for business accounts:

- ❏ Set up accounts.

- ❏ Order checks, deposit slips and bank deposit stamp.

- ❏ Determine need for business credit/debit card.

- ❏ Determine need for Visa/Mastercard servicing account.

❏ Obtain DEA number or change address:

- ❏ Order prescription pads.

❏ Establish electronic tax filing account (EFTPS).

❏ Apply for, or change, malpractice insurance.

❏ Determine method of business accounting:

- ❏ outside sources

- ❑ accountant or bookkeeper

- ❑ business software such as QuickBooks, Peachtree

❑ Determine need to apply for payroll services such as Paychex.

❑ Interview and select printer:

- ❑ determine immediate needs;

- ❑ business cards;

- ❑ letterhead and envelopes;

- ❑ brochures;

- ❑ announcements to colleagues, friends, family.

4. SELLER AND PURCHASER CONFERENCE(S)

❑ Discuss employees' salaries, benefits and bonuses.

❑ Discuss sick day and vacation policies.

❑ Provide/obtain employees' salary histories and work records.

❑ Review fee schedule.

❑ Discuss seller's policies for warranty work.

❑ Discuss seller's policies for pro bono or discounted work.

❑ Obtain/revise/write office policy manual.

❑ Review new patient procedures.

❑ Review case presentation procedures.

❑ Review minimum of 10 patient charts for diagnosis consistency.

❑ Discuss current suppliers and labs.

❑ Discuss specialists used.

❑ Discuss office staff meeting policies/frequency.

❑ Review seller's list of patient charts to be kept (family, friends).

❑ Review seller's ongoing treatments of special needs patients.

5. PRIOR TO CLOSING

❑ Prepare letter of introduction/transfer of practice to patients

    ❑ Seller normally composes.

    ❑ Purchaser revises and approves.

    ❑ Send out immediately after closing.

❑ Prepare letter to referral sources.

❑ Prepare letter to other professionals and specialists.

❑ Send announcements to your friends/family and potential referral sources.

❑ Telephone company—order transfer of service agreement:

    ❑ Verizon (800) 483-50000;

    ❑ AT&T/SBC (800) 499-7928;

    ❑ Notify Yellow Pages of business ownership change.

❑ Apply for transfer of software license(s):

- ❑ dental software

- ❑ business software

- ❑ imaging

- ❑ patient education digital

❑ Contact sign company for name addition/change.

❑ Contact property manager for name addition/change.

❑ Transfer or establish credit card servicing agreement.

❑ Determine need to transfer or establish status with:

- ❑ PPO providers (Delta and Blue Cross)

- ❑ capitation providers

- ❑ Medicaid system

❑ Coordinate transfer of practice health insurance plan.

❑ Order new Message on Hold tape.

6. CONCURRENT WITH AND IMMEDIATELY AFTER CLOSING

❑ Notify professional societies of address change:

- ❑ local, state and national levels

- ❑ other professional societies

❑ Transfer maintenance agreements:

- ❑ computer hardware and software

- ❑ postage meter

     ❑ copy machine

❑ Notify service providers for new accounts:

     ❑ oxygen and nitrous tanks

     ❑ security system

     ❑ waste disposal

     ❑ long-distance carrier

     ❑ dental supply companies

     ❑ office supplies

     ❑ laboratories

     ❑ direct vendors/suppliers

     ❑ display advertising vendors

❑ Determine need for new certificate of occupancy and schedule transfer of utilities with:

     ❑ local city department (for new certificate of occupancy)

     ❑ building inspection

     ❑ gas company

     ❑ electric company

     ❑ city services: water and waste

❑ Change answering machine tape/message.

❑ Meet with new staff to discuss:

     ❑ phone greeting changes

     ❑ scripting language to patients

     ❑ scheduling treatment appointments for seller

❑ handling of accounts receivables/credit balances

❑ Set up state employment office/workforce commission account. This must be done after your first payroll is made.

❑ Convert dental software to new business:

❑ Establish new provider numbers in dental software.

2

START-UP

"The beginning is the most important part of the work."

—PLATO

Your practice is born and now exists legally. You are treating your first patients. Get to know them well. You probably will never forget them.

CHALLENGE

Most young practitioners underestimate money needs and necessary marketing. The main challenge is not to burn through what little cash is available. You need to follow up on cash projections you have given to the bank to see if you are on the right track.

FOCUS

Young practices require establishing a patient base, a reliable delivery system, and a market presence, along with tracking and conserving cash flow.

MONEY SOURCES

Family, friends, suppliers, customers, banks.

THE CHALLENGE OF UNDERESTIMATED MONEY AND MARKETING NEEDS

It is very exciting to be in your very own business. You park your car in your own spot; everyone says, "Good morning, Dr." and hands you your coffee the way you like it—and then stares at you when the first two patients are a no show and the X-ray machine breaks down while in operation.

As Bill Murray said in *Stripes*, "And then reality sets in." Being the boss can be very lonely. You are the man, and you must have answers. Your cash flow projections for the bank are built on ideal conditions, and unfortunately, conditions in a dental practice or any business are rarely ideal. The "infant" stage of your practice is a critical time for cash flow management and marketing—and marketing takes money! A realistic look at the first month of a newly acquired dental practice would look like this:

WEEK 1

MONDAY

Everybody is excited to meet the new doc. The staff is a little nervous and wondering what to do. Patients immediately compare you to old doc and ask how old you are. Two hygiene patients have mouths full of old, breaking fillings and tell you the old doc has been watching them for years and no treatment is necessary. All checks received today are addressed to old doc and must be deposited in his account.

TUESDAY

Receptionist is sick and she is the one who knows how to make the coffee. Hygienist reminds you that she is going on vacation next week as previously arranged with old doc, and wants to know if you will be paying her for those days since she has worked here 12 years.

WEDNESDAY

First bill comes from your accountant. It also has a memo to remind you that the franchise tax report is due on the fifteenth. When seating a bridge prepared by the previous doc, you break porcelain and send back to lab. Deposit today is $242.

THURSDAY

Emergency patient comes in, needs a root canal, and endo system in office is not what you learned in dental school.

FRIDAY

TGIF—only half a day. Catch up on paperwork and correspondence. Everyone has already left office and you don't know where the toner is for copy machine.

WEEK 2

MONDAY

Chairside assistant's baby is sick. Temporary hygienist reeks of smoke (and doesn't know where anything is). Patient who has been with practice 15 years complains about hygienist. Slow collections in weekend mail. Receptionist says Mondays are always slow for collections.

TUESDAY

Chairside assistant is back and likes old doc impression technique better than yours and wants to show you how he did it.

WEDNESDAY

Receptionist wants you to buy Girl Scout cookies from her daughter. Old doc always did. Payday.

THURSDAY

Letter comes in mail from insurance company stating they need you to fill out more forms before you can become their preferred provider, which accounts for 25 percent of your practice.

FRIDAY

You have a margarita at lunch with wife and say, "This is more of a challenge than I thought, but it is going to be great."

WEEK 3

MONDAY

Hygienist returns and tells you she wants to go part-time.

TUESDAY

Collections are very slow. Receptionist says Tuesdays are always slow.

WEDNESDAY

Patient scheduled for four hours and 12 laminates is a no show. Appointment made four months ago. Turns out it was old doc's niece.

THURSDAY

New patient walks in with a bag of four sets of dentures made in the last five years and wants you to make a new set. Haven't we already treated her?

FRIDAY

Wife turns down margarita at lunch and tells you she is pregnant. No margarita for you either. Tequila shot.

WEEK 4

MONDAY

Yes, you know Mondays are always slow collections.

TUESDAY

Receptionist tells you collections will improve if they just had someone else to help answer the phone.

WEDNESDAY

Leak in lab.

THURSDAY

Principal calls from high school next door. Catcher on baseball team broke two front teeth. Parents have no money. Can we help, great kid, prom tomorrow night?

FRIDAY

Payday. Wife tells you she wants to quit her job.

This scenario would really be funny if it weren't the truth. I bought a dental practice in 2004. The day after we closed the deal, I called the office from the airport to see how the first day was going and one-third of the staff had quit. They did not even work one day with me before they quit! As I type this, I am receiving a text from my office telling me the vacuum pump is broken. A dental practice manager needs to be ready for all scenarios, just as a pilot needs to be ready for any type of situation. Anyone can fly an airplane on a calm, sunny day. It is the true success stories that can guide the plane in the storm. It does take a cast-iron stomach.

If this does not seem what you want to sign up for, go back and read the part about associateships. If you are ready for an adventure, have great will for the fight, and the desire to control your own destiny regardless of daily obstacles, continue on. Fortunately, we have steps to focus on to help you on your path to success.

Focus on establishing a patient base, reliable delivery system, and a market presence while tracking and conserving cash flow. An established dental practice, by definition, already has an established patient base.

The focus needs to be on retaining the patients who have been treated in the practice, and expanding on that base. Retaining the patients can be done with internal marketing. Expanding the base will require external marketing.

Internal marketing involves activities that promote your practice within the office. Internal marketing is a powerful way to retain the patients you already have because it focuses on your patients' total experience in the office. It helps build a relationship between you (the new doc) and your patient. Not only is it great for your business but it actually makes your experience richer as you begin to treat people, not just teeth. It can even make you a better dentist. And it is really inexpensive! Internal marketing ideas are only limited by your imagination, so make a game with your staff and get creative.

Here are a few ideas:

- Call your patients at the end of the day to see how they feel after their treatment.

- Send letters to your patient base introducing yourself and your staff.

- Highlight staff retained from old doc.

- Give movie tickets to patients for their referrals.

- Give free teeth whitening for any patient referral.

- Send letters to your patients' physicians, reporting their blood pressure. This is a great idea because you are doing a service for your patient, updating physician records and impressing your patient's physician with your conscientiousness. And it is a door opener for a lunch meeting to tell that physician about how good you are at laminates.

- Send personal thank-you notes to all the patients you see, thanking them for staying with your practice.

- Use patient services whenever possible—good way to build relationship and to network.

I could write a separate book on this subject, but you get the idea.

External marketing is straight advertising. When to use advertising depends on patient flow in the office and staff capability. You should evaluate your ability to deliver great care in a professional manner, both from a dental standpoint and a staff capability standpoint. You don't want to advertise something you may not be able to deliver. Give yourself a few months (a soft opening) to evaluate your staff's ability to efficiently answer the phone, see that patients flow through the office smoothly, and effectively bill and collect. If you are unsatisfied with your staff performance, you have a choice. You can train your staff, or you can change your staff. You will probably need training in running a dental practice yourself. An excellent management training program is Breakaway Practice Seminars at www.breakawaypracticeseminars.com. If you cannot change your staff performance, you must change your staff. Do not external market until you are good at all of these things, because external advertising gives you one shot at the new patient and you don't want to blow it. External marketing, although reasonable for the exposure you get, and certainly necessary for the capable, confident, growing practice, is still costly. Fledgling practices must be frugal. We have worked with an extremely cost-effective dental marketing company called Chrisad. They are the world's oldest and largest dental marketing firm: www.chrisad.com.

Be patient with the process of signing up for insurance plans and acclimating to the new staff. Monitor collections and systems diligently. Don't assume things are getting done. You should be able to have systems in place to collect from insurance companies, collect in pace with cash flow and pay bills on schedule by month three. Until then, you will be burning through your cash, so be very careful about every expense.

MONEY SOURCES

It is time to try to stay away from family and friends for cash in this developmental stage. Your ability to manage your bills and cash flow independently will define you as a businessman. If cash really becomes short, try to negotiate with vendors for leasing options for equipment, more lenient payment options or try to obtain lines of credit at the bank. The start-up of your practice will try your patience and give you great stories to tell your children, but it really is worth it.

3

GROWTH

"Growth is never by mere chance; it is the result of forces working together."

—James Cash Penney

Your practice has made it through the toddler years and is now a child. Production and collections are increasing. Your clinical skills are maturing and you are adding more range to your treatment options. You have many opportunities and issues and must stay abreast of developing situations to continue your upward momentum.

Personally, you are in the family building phase. You are looking for the house you will raise your family in. You might have just bought your first nice car, or maybe a junior membership at the club.

CHALLENGE

The biggest challenge practices face in the growth phase is dealing with ever-increasing demands for time and money. As your schedule gets busier, you must learn to be more efficient from a clinical and delivery standpoint. You must also learn to be efficient from a profitability standpoint. Effective management is required and possibly a new business plan.

FOCUS

Growth life cycle practices are focused on running the practice in a more formal fashion to deal with increased production and collection. Better accounting and management systems will have to be set up. New employees will have to be hired to deal with the influx of new patients.

CHALLENGE OF EVER-INCREASING DEMANDS ON TIME AND MONEY

The growth phase of a dental practice is exciting for the dentist because survival has been achieved. Some predictability in new patient numbers has been achieved. A reasonable confidence in the ability to collect from patients and insurance companies has been attained, and this is a good feeling. With experience, the young practitioner has become more proficient in his dental craft, and even practices with a little bit of a "swagger." He confidently discusses some of his more complex cases at the dental meeting with his friends and is anxious to discuss dentistry with the new dental school graduates, even though they are only three years behind him in experience. He has probably already started a family. A realistic look at a month in the life of a practice in the growth phase would look like this:

WEEK 1

MONDAY

Next-door neighbor called last night with a toothache and wants to be a new patient. Because you want to impress him, you tell him to call the office at 7 a.m. and your office will work with him in the morning. He misunderstands and comes in the office at 7 a.m. At the same time, your biggest nightmare patient also shows up, complaining loudly in the reception area about his crown, which came loose when he ate a gummy bear at the movies the previous evening. He also complains about how expensive you are. (He is the one you gave the senior discount to.) You have a bridge prep scheduled at 7:15 a.m.

TUESDAY

Your office manager, the one who led the way as you moved into your growth stage, your "right hand man," is moving to Wasilla, Alaska, to be a soccer mom and get involved in local politics. She is giving you one month's notice.

WEDNESDAY

You have a huge production day, have to work through lunch, haven't eaten since breakfast, and need to be at girls' basketball practice at 4 p.m. An emergency patient calls at 3:30 p.m. She has broken her front tooth into the pulp and is leaving town tomorrow. You are too exhausted to have an upset stomach. Call wife and she will coach practice. She asks if the girls will need to bring their gloves to practice. You go back to work and become someone's hero.

THURSDAY

Three interviewees for office manager today. The first one has a great resume but has worked for three dentists in last two years, and when asked, she is happy to say what she did not like about her previous employers. The second one has a great resume and a great interview but has salary demands of almost half what the going rate is. Why?

FRIDAY

Normally a half day, then lunch with wife, but today, busy week demands you take time Friday afternoon to catch up.

WEEK 2

MONDAY

Your phone receptionist gives you her resume and wants to apply for office manager position. She is capable and you have already considered her for the position. She has requested $800 more per month than current office manager. She tells you she is going through a divorce and will need more money for living expenses. She tells you she loves working in the office, but if she does not get the job, she will have to leave. You ask yourself if blackmail is legal in your state.

TUESDAY

Extremely busy day; everything was smooth; you are happy with the treatment you provided today; collections were great. You are exhausted and looking forward to dinner, then the couch. Your wife reminds you when you get home that you have parents' night at the school and should be home by 9:30 p.m.

WEDNESDAY

Three more office manager interviews at lunch. Phone receptionist greets them coldly and sneers at you when she "drops" their resumes on your desk.

THURSDAY

Friend of father gets his teeth cleaned. He sees practice appears busy and asks if he can speak privately to you after his visit. In your private office he says, "Doctor, you are really successful now," and he would like you to donate $2500 to his favorite charity. You really are getting successful, but man, that is a lot of money. He has referred a lot of patients to you.

FRIDAY

Lunch with wife who tells you the kids' private school tuition is due and it is $10,500. She says you look a little green.

WEEK 3

MONDAY

Mondays are always awesome. First patient is for endo fill. You are out of gutta-percha. Patient comes out of the bathroom, tells your front desk you are out of toilet paper. Very busy morning. Anterior bonding case needs a certain shade. You have 12 shades but not that one. Your chairside assistant tells you that you should have it. You know you should have it, but you don't. Who is ordering supplies anyway?

TUESDAY

You decide to promote your phone receptionist to replace your office manager. You will give her the raise even though you think it is outrageous, because the candidates you have met are terrible, and if you don't hire her, you are afraid you will have to replace two front-office staff at the same time. Your chairside assistant would like to talk to you to tell you she is upset. She feels you are blaming her for the lack of supplies. You have a great production day and have done beautiful work all day. Your collections are 100 percent for the month and 98 percent for the year. Why do you have a stomachache when you get home?

WEDNESDAY

Great day at work. Five new patients today all want cosmetic treatment. Your office manager tells you at the end of the day that the earliest time they can get in is in five weeks.

THURSDAY

Bank accounts are low after payroll today. Wife tells you her car was making funny noises today and maybe you should start thinking about a new car. Her roommate from college is married to an eye doctor and she just got that new cute Mercedes SUV. Don't you think your family should be safe?

FRIDAY

Very busy Friday morning with great cases. Ready for a restful weekend.

WEEK 4

MONDAY

5:30 a.m. feels like 3:30 a.m. You need a vacation after this weekend. Dinner Friday night with the in-laws. Soccer game at nine Saturday morning.

First birthday party for niece at pizza place with arcade at noon. Noise level is equal to jet engine and you want earplugs. Mow the lawn. You are a doctor and are considering a lawn man. Wedding of frat brother Saturday night. You have to show your college buddies that you still have it and you party 'til 2:00 a.m. You are awakened Sunday morning by the loud sounds of cartoons two hours before you are ready to get out of bed. Brunch at wife's former roommate's house. She wants to show you her new car. But busy weekends don't stop busy Mondays. Full schedule of patients. Living the dream.

TUESDAY

Crown and bridge lab bill in the mail. First, the good news: you did 30 crowns last month. Now, the bad news: your favorite lab is raising fees to over $200. How are you going to afford $6000 worth of lab bills and still accept PPOs?

WEDNESDAY

While in office before lunch, contemplating cost of lab bills and increase in payroll with new office manager situation, hygienist walks in to tell you that she had her biggest production month ever and she would like to talk about a raise or at least a bonus. Four new patients in afternoon tell you, as they leave and make appointments for restorative work, that they love your hygienist.

THURSDAY

Your wife calls you at work to tell you that her best friend has to wait four weeks for next available cleaning appointment. You have had three unfilled hygiene cancellation appointments this morning. Why couldn't her best friend have gotten her teeth cleaned this morning? (You write a note to remember the Maalox with your supply list.)

FRIDAY

Really busy morning, thank goodness, because you need the money to pay the lab bill and payroll increases...

Being "busy" in our practice has been all of our dreams since the seed stage. When patients see a busy practice, they automatically assume that money is growing on our trees. Staff members worry about their own bills, not ours. Insurance companies worry about their own bottom lines and don't care about our expensive labs (or our patients/ their customers!)

Practices in the growth phase have growing pains. Growing pains can be devastating if not managed properly. We work in a very tight margin industry. It is essential to run a dental practice efficiently. Being "busy" can take the soul out of a solo practitioner, as there is only one of him and life and work have so much for him to do. Systems need to be implemented to take much of the load off the dentist and delegate it so that the dentist can sleep at night, knowing things are being taken care of. Inventory must be managed to prevent situations in which the necessary supplies are missing when the patient is already in the chair. Human resource issues need to be consistent to prevent random staff demands. We should be happy to be charitable in our community because it is a good thing to do and also brings us patients. However, it should be part of the budget. We should have goals and expectations of all our staff members in alignment with our goals and expectations. This alignment should be accompanied by intensive training to teach us all to achieve our goals. Now that we know our challenges, let's get started with solutions.

FOCUS

It is very important to begin to run the practice in a more formal fashion. In the start-up phase, the attitude is that everyone pitches in, in all aspects of the practice. In a small office it is easy to see how hard everyone is working. In the growth phase, it is easy for employees to "hide" and everyone starts to assume that someone else is doing a particular task. It won't become apparent until it presents itself in front of the dentist—for example, a lack of supplies for the patient in the chair. Accountability needs to be institutional. When all staff members know what is expected of them and how to do it, the dentist is relieved of time and pressure constraints and life can be worth living again!

Every dental office needs to have:

- ❑ a staff policy manual

- ❑ a staff training manual

- ❑ accounting and bookkeeping systems systematically monitored

The purpose of a staff policy manual is to spell out in black and white specific policies of the practice in order to avoid ambiguity or any miscommunication regarding all issues pertaining to employees and the treatment and care of patients. It should include but not be limited to the following:

❑ Practice name

❑ Mission statement or practice philosophy

❑ Employment policies including:

- ❑ employee selection process

- ❑ at-will employment

- ❑ equal opportunity employment

- ❑ accommodation for disabilities

- ❑ nondiscrimination

- ❑ immigration law compliance/form I-9 requirement

- ❑ code of conduct
- ❑ business ethics
- ❑ nondisclosure
- ❑ non-compete agreement
- ❑ bonding requirements
- ❑ nepotism
- ❑ harassment policy, reporting procedure, investigative process
- ❑ discrimination policy, reporting procedure, investigation process
- ❑ drugs and alcohol/drug testing
- ❑ privacy expectations
- ❑ monitoring of e-mail, computer use, telephone
- ❑ video surveillance
- ❑ disclaimers

❑ Employment status and records including:

- ❑ employment classifications
- ❑ definitions of employee status
- ❑ definition of employee
- ❑ exempt and nonexempt employee
- ❑ part-time and full-time
- ❑ temporary and contract workers
- ❑ background checks
- ❑ education

- ❏ licenses/credentials
- ❏ CPR certification
- ❏ criminal records
- ❏ credit investigation
- ❏ employment and reference checks
- ❏ vaccines
- ❏ outside employment
- ❏ new employee orientation
- ❏ probationary period
- ❏ personnel records: access, changes, medical
- ❏ performance reviews
- ❏ conflict resolution
- ❏ compliance procedures
- ❏ disciplinary warnings
- ❏ progressive discipline
- ❏ separation of employment/resignation/voluntary and involuntary termination
- ❏ severance
- ❏ benefits
- ❏ exit interview
- ❏ returning office property
- ❏ final paycheck
- ❏ former employees
- ❏ post employment inquiries

- ❑ Working Hours
  - ❑ normal working hours
  - ❑ recording of time worked
  - ❑ overtime
  - ❑ on call
  - ❑ attendance
  - ❑ tardiness
  - ❑ absenteeism
  - ❑ breaks/lunch
  - ❑ staff meetings
  - ❑ closure due to weather or emergency
  - ❑ low need time

- ❑ Compensation
  - ❑ payday schedule
  - ❑ basis for determining pay
  - ❑ salary review and raise request policies
  - ❑ time records
  - ❑ payroll deductions
  - ❑ paycheck distribution
  - ❑ direct deposit
  - ❑ errors in pay
  - ❑ loss of paycheck
  - ❑ payroll advances
  - ❑ expense reimbursement

❑ wage garnishments

❑ benefits eligibility

❑ Benefits

❑ medical insurance

❑ dental benefits

❑ vision

❑ life insurance

❑ disability insurance

❑ retirement plan

❑ profit sharing plan

❑ continuing education policies

❑ uniform allowance

❑ bonus system

❑ COBRA coverage

❑ government mandated benefits

❑ Social Security

❑ Medicare

❑ workers compensation

❑ unemployment insurance

❑ Time Off

❑ paid holidays

❑ unpaid/paid personal time

❑ vacation policies

- ❑ sick leave
- ❑ disability leave
- ❑ maternity leave
- ❑ family leave
- ❑ funeral/bereavement leave
- ❑ religious accommodation
- ❑ military leave
- ❑ extended personal leave
- ❑ requesting time off

❑ Workplace standards of conduct

- ❑ job description and expectations
- ❑ what employees can expect from office and vice versa
- ❑ customer relations
- ❑ personal appearance
- ❑ dress code
- ❑ personal hygiene
- ❑ pets
- ❑ office romances
- ❑ parking
- ❑ breast-feeding policy
- ❑ smoking policy
- ❑ use of equipment and supplies policies
- ❑ after hours policy
- ❑ information technology policies

❑ cell phone use

❑ Safety and security

    ❑ OSHA compliance

    ❑ HIPAA compliance

    ❑ workplace violence/weapons

    ❑ building security

    ❑ personal belongings

    ❑ reporting injuries

❑ Signature page

    ❑ acknowledgement of receipt of employee handbook

(Courtesy Randall Otterholt, D.D.S.)

As you can see this covers everything including the kitchen sink. And that is the beauty of it. Every time a situation arises, such as "Can I have a raise?" or "Do we get paid for the day after Thanksgiving?" you simply refer to the manual. If someone dresses inappropriately, instead of an awkward moment, refer to the manual. If someone's gum chewing is driving you mad, ask that person to read the manual that he/she agreed to abide by. If supplies are not stocked, resulting in inability to provide treatment, simply look in the manual to see who is responsible. By not having to get involved in all of these real-life situations, you cover yourself legally, and you reduce strain on yourself both personally and professionally. A start-up practice would obviously benefit from a staff policy manual. A growth practice cannot survive without one.

The purpose of a staff-training manual is to give all employees the tools to perform their expected job duties. Too often, because the dentist is extensively trained for his job duties, we assume that everyone else is equally as trained. This reasoning can be problematic for a few reasons. First, even trained and experienced staff members need to be indoctrinated in the methods used in our own practice. Second, we all understand what the word "assume" stands for and assuming something is being done causes nothing to be done. I "assumed" Jane had cleaned the operatory before the patient was seated. I "assumed" Mary had ordered the endo kit. I "assumed" my assistant had pulled the cord before the impression was taken …

Thirdly, efficient training of staff allows us to mold less-experienced personnel into excellent employees, and homegrown "talent" is less expensive than recruiting experienced employees. Think of the New York Yankee payroll and the free agent market method they employ as opposed to the Oakland Athletic payroll and the "Billy Ball" method they use. Concise training methods are excellent for profitability.

A training manual should include all job descriptions, who is assigned to each task and who is delegated for the task if the assigned staff member is not present (a backup).

It should be very precise and detailed—for example, six heaping scoops of coffee for six cups of coffee.

A useful training manual will include but not be limited to:

- ❏ telephone training
- ❏ answers for patient clinical questions
- ❏ payment option policy
- ❏ appointment book management
- ❏ insurance/collection protocol
- ❏ training on "flowing" patients through the office "handoffs"

- ❏ clinical tray setups for each procedure, with pictures
- ❏ clinical room setups
- ❏ supply list/inventory protocol
- ❏ lab communication protocol

The staff can create the manual. It is simple to do. At a staff meeting have everyone agree to write a list of all the tasks in the office. The list will be longer than the basic one I have included above. Assign and agree on who is responsible for each task. Have the responsible parties write instructions on how these tasks are performed on an individual sheet of paper. This will probably take supervision and guidance from the dentist. After completion, compile the individual sheets, with the job descriptions, instructions, and responsible parties (and backups) into a bound manual, with a directory of employees/backups matched to job descriptions in the front for easy reference.

Simple, right? It is simple, but very time consuming, and we are trying to save time and money in the growth phase. We used this manual building approach after studying practice management with Dr. Scott Leune, DDS at www.breakawaypracticeseminars.com. Breakaway is excellent and would be useful in any phase of the practice cycle.

Although we found the approach great, the implementation was time consuming and we discovered an easier, more efficient way to build the manual and manage many other aspects of the practice. Stratus Dental (www.stratusdental.com) is a practice management company that uses the Internet to automate systems, including training and policy manuals, in the office. It implements many of the useful tools online, leaving the dentist and staff with more time to do the jobs we were trained to do and to live the life we desired. Breakaway and Stratus have been game changers in our practices. They will "formalize" your practice for you.

Accounting and bookkeeping systems need to be monitored on a regular basis. Monthly is optimal, quarterly at the least.

It is very useful if the dentist has a basic understanding of:

- ❏ profit and loss statements and useful percentage guidelines for an efficient profitable practice
- ❏ balance sheets
- ❏ Quick Books or equivalent bookkeeping system
- ❏ tax ramifications regarding the dental practice (helpful when planning a strategy for purchases)

General reading and listening at parties can be a guide for the dentist who probably has a science degree. Let's face it, most of us were chemistry nerds and are not subscribers to *The Wall Street Journal*. It is important in the growth phase to start broadening our business horizons and becoming aware of the environment in which we work. Go to the bookstore on a Saturday morning and go to the business or management section and buy a handful of books. Scan through them and pick ones that are interesting. Some suggestions are *Good to Great* by Jim Collins and *The E-Myth* by Michael Gerber. Look for opportunities for business education advancement. For example, Texas Tech University offers an MBA program specifically for dental practice management. There are many useful tools online. We recommend and are accredited by the Association of Accredited Small Business Consultants (AASBC). It has online (and hard copy) training manuals, including videos and testing for accreditation. The accreditation requires study but it's well worth it to give you all the tools necessary to run the small but *rapidly* growing business you now own. If we are smart enough to get into and out of dental school, we are smart enough to begin to master our own business. You are really stepping up your game!

4

ESTABLISHED

*"Organization isn't about perfection; it's about efficiency,
reducing stress and clutter, saving time and money
and improving your overall quality of life."*

—CHRISTINA SCALISE

Your practice has now matured and is thriving with many loyal patients and a developed niche in the market. The practice is still growing but not explosive. The practice of dentistry has become routine. At continuing education meetings, it becomes more challenging to learn something, because you have learned most of this before. You are active in charities, boards and organizations. You live in the house you dreamed about in dental school. You worry about your handicap and know it would be lower if you could practice more, but you have so much to do with coaching the kids and charity work. You really feel you have arrived.

CHALLENGE

It is far too easy to rest on your laurels during this life stage. You have worked hard and have earned a rest, but the marketplace is relentless and competitive. Stay focused on the big picture. Issues such as the economy, competitors, or changing patient tastes can threaten you.

FOCUS

An established practice should be focused on improvement and productivity. To compete in an established market, you will require better business practices, along with more automation and outsourcing/ insourcing to improve productivity.

MONEY SOURCES

- ❑ banks
- ❑ investors
- ❑ government
- ❑ profits

THE CHALLENGE OF RESTING ON YOUR LAURELS

The establishment phase of a dental practice gives the dentist a chance to reflect on accomplishments, acknowledge successes and failures, contemplate the future. A realistic look at a month in the life of a practice in the established phase would look like this:

WEEK 1

MONDAY

Wife gets up early to prepare your breakfast at the start of the week. Your son scored a touchdown in the game Friday night and the team won. Great weekend! Your wife tells you, after she gets the kids off to school, she has yoga at 9:00 a.m., nail appointment at 11:00 a.m., and she is taking your daughter to get a prom dress after school. You go into the garage to get the car to go to work. You look at your wife's Suburban and happily think of the car trip to Mount Rushmore last summer. You look at your Jag and think you really didn't need to spend the money, but you have worked hard and your friend at the club really got you a great deal. You drive to work without a care in the world. Your office manager has everything in control, the staff is a well-oiled machine and you put on the cruise control.

TUESDAY

Celebration lunch today. Your chairside assistant is celebrating her tenth anniversary in the office. You barely can remember practicing without her. She knows the procedures better than you do and her efficiency and your teamwork can stun you. If you put your hand out, she will put the correct instrument in it even if you don't know what instrument you want yet.

WEDNESDAY

You are happy today because you only have a half day. Tee time at 1:12 p.m.

THURSDAY

Lunch with your endodontist today. After reviewing a few cases, he asks you if you noticed the large dental clinic being built down the street.

FRIDAY

Very successful implant surgery. You are really getting good at this. Wouldn't it be great if you didn't have to waste time doing fillings and could concentrate on the procedures you really enjoy?

WEEK 2

MONDAY

New patient referred to you for implant placement and immediate dentures. Wants to get started right away. Earliest available long appointment is five weeks away.

TUESDAY

Dr. Jones, your dental school classmate, tells you his CEREC machine has changed his life.

WEDNESDAY

Golf is cancelled today because you have previously scheduled a large case in the oral surgeon's office.

THURSDAY

Busy day, but staff is so smooth you are almost bored.

FRIDAY

Continuing ed. You leave at noon. You think that you should be teaching these things.

WEEK 3

MONDAY

You are first one in the office this morning. You notice new patient numbers are steady but stagnant. It isn't really affecting you, because client retention is good.

TUESDAY

Fillings all morning bore you. A new patient in the afternoon asks you if she has to wear a "temporary" when you tell her that her fractured tooth should be treated with a crown. Mental note to self, "Call rep about CEREC demo."

WEDNESDAY

You cannot be more productive and efficient this morning. It is a perfect day. Your golf partner gets to your office at 11:00 a.m. and reads magazines for an hour before you have finished working and are able to join him for lunch and golf. He is early because he has nothing to do. Why does he have so much more money than you do and he doesn't even have to work?

THURSDAY

Demo in morning for CEREC. Crown and bridge lab is expensive and it might be fun to learn how to use the CEREC. You call your accountant in the afternoon to see if it is eligible for a Section 179 deduction.

FRIDAY

Office lease is coming due. You are meeting with real estate agent and landlord at 1:00 p.m. to negotiate new lease. Real estate agent wants to show you buildings for sale, afterward. Do you really want to buy a building?

WEEK 4

MONDAY

Dental school classmate calls to tell you the endo microscope he just bought has changed his life. He also tells you he just got an associate. Frees him up to do the things he likes to do. Double-changed his life. You liked your life! You don't have a CEREC; you don't have an endo microscope; you don't own your own building; and you don't have an associate. Why do you feel so backward?

TUESDAY

Dental school classmate called and said his new superlaser changed his life (just kidding). His divorce really changed his life, but that is another story.

WEDNESDAY

Shot 79 today. Why do I want to change my life?

THURSDAY

Letter in mail from large dental corporation. Wants to know if I am interested in selling my practice. Must be full moon.

FRIDAY

You have a great idea. Not only will you buy a CEREC, you will also buy an endo microscope, a superlaser, and a building to put them in. You will also hire an associate to use them. Ready or not, you are going to change your life. You are not going to get divorced, but you are going to accept change. The only thing that is constant is change.

FOCUS OF IMPROVEMENT AND PRODUCTIVITY

In the growth phase it is easy to stay motivated because successes come rapidly, and it is exciting to "ride on top of the wave." In the established phase, motivation is harder to maintain because of the routine. *Motivation must be attained by constant improvement and more productivity.* This is because even though a great level of success has been achieved, in the market place, you must continue to improve just to stay even, much less gain on the competition. Motivation can also be attained through fear: of losing status achieved, losing things we have, and the ability to be charitable to those we love and to great causes. Fear can be the greatest motivator.

Improvements in practice implementation and productivity can be achieved by outsourcing/insourcing and automation.

Outsourcing is the contracting out of a business process to a third party. In a dental practice it can include:

❏ Using outside payroll services/even contracting a company to hire your staff for the purpose of improved benefits and less costly human resource solutions;

❏ Hiring outside marketing/social media;

❏ Hiring outside bookkeeping services;

❏ Outside laboratory (standard, not the exception);

❏ Associate dentists;

❏ Contracting specialists to work in-house.

Insourcing is the cessation of contracting a business function and the commencement of performing it internally. In a dental practice it can include having an in-house lab. How convenient would it be to have your own lab?

Hiring outside payroll, marketing, and bookkeeping services are very handy and efficient ways to help the practice focus on what actually makes it thrive. As a dentist, you waste time and energy, stewing over a computer after hours. It is the equivalent of your accountant fixing his own teeth: bad for business, bad for relationships. Unless you have an extensive background in a certain subject, let the professionals step in. Have your advisor team help you with a strategy for outsourcing business services.

Outside dental labs are a standard. Most dentists today are not as trained as the old-school dentists who used to do a lot more lab work in dental school and never considered making their own crowns (unless they owned a CEREC). Consider the amount of time it would take out of a productive day if you were sitting at a bench making each crown—and the revenue lost.

Now consider how much more productive you could be with an associate working for you, or having a CEREC machine. Also, consider how many patients you refer to specialists. What would treating all of those referred patients in your office do for your bottom line?

Before you become overwhelmed with the prospects of having an associate, CEREC machine, in-house lab, or other "life changers," stop and consider the pros and cons.

CEREC (chairside economical restoration of esthetic ceramics) allows a dentist to produce an indirect ceramic dental restoration, using a variety of computer-assisted technologies, including 3D photography and CAD/CAM. The benefits are that restorations can be performed in a single visit, no "temporary" necessary, and for a reduced lab fee. The drawbacks to CEREC are initial cost, learning curve before successful implementation can be achieved with consistency, and esthetics.

CEREC is just one example of cutting-edge, life-changing technology that is constantly being put in front of dentists. It is an excellent product that can be used very successfully by skilled operators.

Before buying a CEREC or any piece of technology, ask yourself these questions:

❑ How long will it take to get my return on investment?

❑ Will it, and how will it, attract patients to me? (Ask this question 12 times and don't ask the sales rep.)

❑ Am I willing to make the time commitment to use it effectively? (Or am I going to use it as a clothes hanger, like the treadmill in my bedroom?)

❑ What will be the benefits to my patients?

DO YOU NEED YOUR OWN LABORATORY?

You should consider an in-house laboratory if your purpose is more control over quality, convenient custom shading, very close communication with your technician, and a high volume of "large case" crown and bridge in the practice. If your purpose is to save lab fees or have less hassle, you should reconsider. The cost of space used in the office, cost of supplies, cost of technician—all of that becomes a fixed, not a variable, cost and could make owning your own dental lab the kind of "life changer" you may not want.

ARE YOU READY FOR AN ASSOCIATE?

Why do you want one? Adding an associate to an established dental practice is a different strategy from having associates in an expansion practice, as you will learn in the next chapter. Dentists in established practices generally consider adding associates for the following reasons:

• Relieve "busy-ness" (missing golf on Wednesday afternoon is problematic);

- Relieve pressure of having to do everything yourself;

- Do procedures you don't like doing, freeing yourself up for procedures you enjoy;

- Attract more patients.

These are all emotional issues. A decision to add an associate is best made unemotionally. Sally McKenzie (www.mckenziemgmt.com) has two excellent rules to follow before adding an associate:

Rule #1: Measure the number of truly "active" patients. See formula at www.mckenziemgmt.com.

Rule #2: Be sure clinical efficiencies cannot be improved to resolve the perceived reasons an associate is desired in the first place.

The dentist needs to understand that associates are a drain on an established practice that needs to have resources, not provide them. Associates require many more exposures to new patients than the established senior dentist. Their skills may not be as broad, their diagnostic abilities and case presentation skills not as developed, credibility with older patients lessened, and speed in treatment slower. Because so many more patients are often needed to "feed" an associate, marketing expenses will have to increase to keep even. The senior dentist, also, is often hesitant to give the "good" patients to the associate and the effect is that the senior doc is working just to support the associate. If the senior doc only gives the "trash" work to the associate, the associate becomes unhappy. All of this is not the type of "life change" desired.

Perhaps a better way to add production to an established practice is to contract a specialist to come into the office to provide specialty treatment in-house. Oral surgery, endo, perio and even ortho can be provided at a great convenience to your patients. Many specialists are looking for ways to augment their incomes by working in general practices. Typically, the general practice makes the appointments, collects fees and pays the specialist. It can happen on Wednesday afternoon when you are golfing!

The moral of the story is an established practice needs twice as many patients as it can handle before it should add an associate, and that would put it in the expansion phase.

5

EXPANSION

"Life begins where your comfort zone ends."

—Neale Donald Walsch

This life cycle is characterized by a new period of growth in the practice or perhaps the addition of practices. This stage is often the choice of the dentist to gain a larger patient pool and expand opportunities.

Dentists evolving from the established phase make a personal decision to continue into the expansion phase, or to skip it completely and move into the mature phase. This decision is based on the dentist's nature and his satisfaction with the practice of dentistry. Many dentists love the act of fixing teeth and never tire of it. They can never quench their thirst to learn and their passion for dentistry increases rather than decreases over time. If their monetary needs are still great, they must be satisfied by shrewd investments, frugal shopping habits, and the virtue of patience, because no amount of money can provide the joy given to them by dentistry. Many dentists, however, tire of the daily hard work of dentistry. Their backs begin to hurt. They have accomplished everything they feel important in their dental careers as practitioners, and their entrepreneurial spirit leads them to search for more challenges. They know the answer to the question of why their golfing buddies seem so much more successful than they do and don't even work.

CHALLENGE

Moving into new markets requires the planning and research of a seed or start-up practice. Focus should be on businesses or practices that complement your existing experience and capabilities. Getting into businesses unrelated to what you know can cause you to lose everything you have worked so hard for.

FOCUS

Add new products or services to existing practice or expand with more practices in more markets.

MONEY SOURCES

Joint ventures, banks, investors.

CHALLENGE OF NEW GROWTH IN EXISTING PRACTICE AND ADDITION OF NEW OFFICES

You are looking for new opportunities and directions. You are not content to move into the mature phase of your practice life cycle. You see dentistry as an opportunity and your adventurous side is taking over. Although you are tiring of being chair-bound, you are not ready to slow down. You are interested in business and want to expand the only business you truly know. A realistic look at a month in the life of a practice in the expansion phase would look like this:

WEEK 1

MONDAY

You come into the office late today because you have just returned from Italy and you are jet lagged. You have a meeting with your office manager to review the last month. You have been receiving daily computer updates on your iPad regarding production and collection, new patients, bank balances, and work scheduled to be performed, but you are still interested to see what is happening in the office in person. You catch up on the news on who has been out sick, who is leaving on vacation, and you review large case photos completed with your associates. They didn't even miss you and you don't know if this makes you happy or sad.

TUESDAY

Meeting with accountant in morning and stockbroker in afternoon.

WEDNESDAY

Full mouth extraction case in morning. You feel so lucky that you get to do the work that you enjoy when you want to but don't have to keep a full schedule.

THURSDAY

Conference call with your team from Stratus dental (www. stratusdental.com) to discuss your participation in the leadership bootcamp.

FRIDAY

Daughter and her husband are coming to town for the weekend

WEEK 2

MONDAY

Visiting all the offices this week. First stop at 6:45 a.m. to evaluate efficiency in the huddle. Trying to make them shorter. Afterward, you sit with one of your newest associates to discuss case presentation and you also sit in the chair with him to demonstrate endo system. Review production and collection progress with the office manager and go over staff evaluations to be presented that week. Lunch with senior associate in office number two. She is frustrated with her lack of control of the office scheduling process. You discuss possible solutions but don't really solve her concerns. She is a great dentist and you want her happy. You have a stomach-ache after lunch.

TUESDAY

Same routine as Monday. Senior associate in office number three wants to consider a different crown and bridge lab. Office manager in office number four is going on maternity leave, and the compressor in office number five needs replacing at a cost of $18,000.

WEDNESDAY

Meeting with Stratus Dental regarding marketing ROI.

THURSDAY

All work from home today. Internet and computerized reports make daily office visits unnecessary. Phone conversations with all the offices. Things are smooth.

FRIDAY

Golf and massage.

WEEK 3

MONDAY

Meeting with a broker about a practice recently listed that fits the prototype of what you like to buy.

TUESDAY

List of all the repairs needed in all the offices comes to your desk. You spend the morning on the phone with supply houses, repairmen, and your contractor. It is always something.

WEDNESDAY

You sit in on staff evaluations. They are productive and positive. You follow a format that helps with communication of office expectations and the staff seems to respond.

THURSDAY

You visit the office listed for sale on Monday and like it. Work now begins to perform due diligence to try to make the purchase possible and develop staff.

FRIDAY

Phone calls with accountant to prepare financials, Stratus Dental (www.stratusdental.com) to begin staffing search, and bookkeeper to review bills. You are thrilled that you no longer *have* to fix teeth for a living. People think you are retired. They don't realize that you work very hard at not working.

WEEK 4

MONDAY

Office number five is not performing as projected. (Note to self to visit office number five to review systems and training.)

TUESDAY

Interviewing potential associates. Were you ever that young?

WEDNESDAY

All offices convene for full day of OSHA training. It is a great opportunity for all the office staffs to meet and share experiences. You can't believe how many people are there.

THURSDAY

Meeting with insurance agent and human resources coordinator. What is the Affordable Care Act going to do for our health care costs? (Note to self to re-review personnel manual.)

FRIDAY

Packing for convention. Need to stay abreast with not only dental education but also our changing industry.

The expansion phase of the life cycle is very stimulating because you are constantly involved in new, exciting tasks. Every day is different. You are never bored because you are learning and reading and studying different aspects of our "business" of dentistry. You realize how physically difficult being a dentist can be, and you almost feel guilty that you can earn a great living and provide a great service without all the physical wear and tear on your body. Opportunities to provide dental care were always limited by the amount of dental work you could actually perform. You no longer have limits, and it feels good. You are back in control of your time, in control of your interests, and you have regained your passion. You are heavily invested in your business. There are no guarantees, but your future is in your own hands and you are going for it.

FOCUS ON ADDING NEW PRODUCTS OR SERVICES TO EXISTING PRACTICES, OR EXPANSION

Dental practices, like all businesses, expand for the purpose of providing more services and creating profit. Our motivation in the expansion of our dental practice has changed from being a solo practitioner and independently delivering dentistry and practicing our craft to owning a practice with dentist associates, supported by large staffs, who now provide the dental care, with expanded specialty treatment available, more convenient and accessible hours, and a vast array of products and services not possible for a solo practitioner. The owner-dentist has changed from a main focus on being a craftsman/artisan /doctor to being a leader/visionary. As Michael Gerber, author of *The E-Myth* might say, "The solo dentist owns a job; the owner of an expansion practice owns a business."

Before starting on the expansion phase, which could amount to starting a second career, it is important to consider why you want to do this. The obvious, easy answer is "To make more money." This answer is too simplistic and rarely leads to a successful outcome. Money for greed and "scorekeeping" can lead to shortcuts, which are bad in any business, but unethical, immoral, and dangerous in our healthcare industry. We have taken an oath to provide the best dental care possible and expanded practices truly are an exceptional opportunity to give our patients *better*, more convenient, and more economical treatment. Expansion without high-quality care will be disaster by the power of ten for the owner-dentist, financially and ethically.

Good reasons for expansion would include:

- Providing quality care in underserved areas;

- Bringing specialty or cosmetic services to areas previously without access;

- Twice the amount of patients in the practice than the solo dentist can serve as previously discussed in the established phase;

- Desire to build an efficient more cost effective organization/business model;

- Provide a platform to compete against a marketplace already being deluged by corporate dentistry;

- Provide charitable opportunities.

Having laudable purposes for expanding your already excellent practice will make it easier for your established existing staff to understand and follow your vision. Although you will be purposefully adding many more employees, you will need and want the people who got you to this juncture to continue the journey with you, for your sake and theirs. They are the backbone and soul of your organization and to grow without your soul will be counterproductive to your purpose. They convey all the positive attributes that you want to impart to the new staff.

Once you and your crew commits to an expansionist vision, the fun begins. You will focus on many of the same steps that you focused on in the seed stage, and you will face many similar challenges. You will face the challenge of market acceptance and pursuit of a niche. You will address the challenge differently than you did in the seed stage because you already have a niche established. Different from the seed and start-up stage when you are at ground zero, have no patients, no culture, no brand, the expansion phase gives you the great benefit of having a culture, a brand and identity already established. The challenge of market acceptance will be more easily overcome after you face the expansion practice challenge of giving your talents, your soul, and your vision to multiples of people, not just to yourself and your immediate staff. In *The E-Myth*, Michael Gerber discusses Ray Kroc visiting the McDonald brothers' hamburger stand and thinking what a great business it could be. Kroc did not focus on making hamburgers; he *focused on systems* to make billions of great hamburgers! In the expansion phase, your product has already been developed. Consider your dental practice as the product. Now *focus on systems* to deliver your dental culture, brand, and excellent service. Simple, right?

It can be if you can overcome the feelings of having to do everything yourself, if you want something done right you must do it yourself, or the feeling that you are indispensable. If you can overcome your own *ego*, then, with good marketing and systems to train you to provide sustained excellence at all levels, and good location selection, you will have no boundaries.

If you cannot get over your own ego, if you are committed to the idea that no one you could ever hire could get crowns as good as yours, building a great organization will be difficult. Henry Ford did not build every car on his own. Papa John doesn't bake every pizza. Steven Jobs didn't build every computer, and Warren Buffett lets his staff help with investments. If they can let go, so can you.

Once you let go, there are many different ways to build your organization. It will be necessary, however, to follow some basic tenets.

First, read *The E-Myth* by Michael Gerber. He will discuss in detail the principles of working on your business, not in it. He discusses the "the franchise prototype," and the concept that successful businesses should be replicable. After all, aren't expansion practices trying to clone the culture, the identity, the soul of the "prototype" practice you and your dedicated staff have established? Michael Gerber explains the rules that must be followed for "the franchise prototype" including:

a) Consistent, exceptional value to customers (patients), employees, suppliers, and lenders;

b) The model will be operated by people with the least possible skill level, not the highest;

c) Impeccable order;

d) Operations manuals;

e) Uniform, predictable service and dress.

Second, decide on a business structure, including corporate structure and organizational structure. These will once again be topics to discuss with your already-assembled, professional advisor team, including your lawyer and accountant. However, the expansion of your practice will require another layer of professional advice.

Management, real estate, human resources, marketing, insurance, and understanding of the marketplace all are issues that are the order of the day and will require research, diligence, and imagination. The owner-dentist can gain management advice from excellent sources such as Breakaway (www.breakawaypracticeseminars.com), and great marketing advice from Chrisad Dental Marketing, the world's oldest and largest dental marketing company (www.chrisad.com). Human resources for the dental practice and insurance updates for the ever-changing landscape of payments should be constantly researched online, or at study groups, or at dental meetings.

If your passion is constant reading, studying, and meetings, you can find all your answers on your own. It will consume most of your time and could take away some of your freedom for opportunities that was one of the goals of expansion in the first place.

Another way to approach management, human resources, and so on, is through companies such as Stratus Dental (www.stratusdental.com). Stratus is an innovative, dental management services company focused on providing leading, independent, private dental practices a way to preserve their independence and thrive in the midst of industry consolidation, a saturated marketplace, and a multitude of daily operational issues, including reduced reimbursements. These objectives are obtained by online interface with the individual offices, staff training, individual market studies and individual accountability. If you are the type of person who wants to know how the clock is built, and are passionate about how the process works, do all the research and background work yourself. If you are the kind of person who is only interested in what time it is, and the end result, rather than the journey, consider Stratus Dental (www.stratusdental.com).

Third, remember, remember, remember, that your job is to lead the group to provide great dentistry (lots of great dentistry), not to perform all the dentistry yourself.

Money sources creative and opportunistic financing options with exceptional investor value. Once you have done your due diligence in forming your organization, have created systems that can be originated in your prototype established practice with demonstrable success and replicated in others, you can build proformas of future performance to lenders, and your options for loans will be surprisingly different from when you were in the seed or start-up phase. You may self-finance your expansion, or seek banks or outside investors. Your comfort level will determine how fast you expand. If you start slowly, adding one practice at a time, you can play it close to the vest and borrow money conservatively. If you expand on a larger scale, you probably will need outside investors. Venture investors will be interested in your expansion if your research is well documented, if your prototype practice has had good net returns, and if you have well-documented systems in place to replicate your prototype. Go for it!

6

MATURE

"The purpose of life is to fight maturity."

—DICK WERTHIMER

The last two chapters are the hardest chapters for me to write. I have difficulty considering the ramifications of being a certain age and having the feeling that there is nothing left for me to do. For this reason, the mature phase and the exit phase are hypothetical stages only and should be thought of merely as that.

Year after year, sales and profits tend to be stable. However, competition remains fierce. Eventually, production begins to decrease and a decision is needed whether to expand or exit.

CHALLENGE

Practices in the mature phase will be challenged with dropping production, profits, and negative cash flow. Ask if it is time to return to the expansion phase or move on to the final life-cycle stage: exit.

FOCUS

Search for new opportunities and business ventures. Cutting costs and finding ways to sustain cash flow are vital to the mature phase.

MONEY SOURCES

Suppliers, owners, banks.

CHALLENGE OF DROPPING PRODUCTION, PROFITS AND NEGATIVE CASH FLOW

This is the problem I have with the mature phase. Why would you want to be in a phase of dropping production, profits, and negative income? That is why the mature phase is hypothetical. Instead of discussing ways to deal with all the bad things, let's talk about all the good things that can happen if you don't let your practice become mature. Years ago, at a practice seminar, someone asked what he should do if he suffered a down month. The speaker replied, "Don't have a down month!" I agree. In boxing, the adage is a good offense beats a good defense. Keep throwing punches. My advice is to skip the mature phase. Keep throwing punches. Go directly from expansion to exit. And only go when you are ready.

SEARCH FOR NEW OPPORTUNITIES AND VENTURES

Now we are back on a subject I am interested in: expansion. When we left off in expansion, we were following the rules of "the franchise prototype." With Michael Gerber's vision of business building the implementation of systems in your office by Stratus Dental (www.stratusdental.com), pointed marketing, shrewd real estate usage, and strong visionary leadership, your practice is exceeding your wildest dental school dreams. You have every "thing" you could possibly need. Your children's education is paid for. You have traveled. You have stimulated yourself by building an organization. You have associates you are proud of. Now what?

Why do you want to expand? What motivation do you have to keep pushing forward, and the bigger question: what motivates the already very accomplished? The question of when and why to expand can be looked at from a purely business analytic but should be looked at from a personal and psychological perspective. It's good to look at it from a human perspective because, once again, we must remember the morality and the ethics involved in our dental profession and also, the ability to lead is made a lot easier with clarity of motive.

Obviously, the scope of this book is not a psychology text, but at this career stage, psychology should be considered. As we have progressed through the different life-cycle stages of a dental practice, I have tried to give a realistic vision of what a dentist's real life could be as well as his practice life. I try to illustrate this through "typical months in the life-cycle stage" vignettes. This is to give you a framework of why certain decisions are made, or why certain attitudes are adopted. It also is to give you a basic timeline showing when certain phases are likely to occur. Most decisions or attitudes from seed to establishment are in response to outside stimuli, a reaction to the basic needs of you and your family. The need to pay student loans, the need to buy a house, pay for school, cars, finance a practice, and so on. As you progress through the establishment phase into expansion, many of your choices become more optional. It is also a period when one has more time for reflection.

Maslow's hierarchy of needs, delivered in his 1943 paper "A Theory of Human Motivation," is illustrated by a pyramid with the more basic needs at the bottom. The needs from the bottom to the top are:

- **Physiological:** breathing, food, water, sex, sleep, homeostasis, excretion

- **Safety of:** body, employment, resources, morality, family health, property

- **Love/belonging:** friendship, family, intimacy

- **Esteem/self esteem:** confidence, achievement, respect of others and respect by others

- **Self-actualization:** morality, creativity, spontaneity, problem solving, lack of prejudice, acceptance of facts

If you draw parallels with the "seven life cycles of a dental practice," all needs except self-actualization are met by the established stage. The time of expansion and extended successful expansion are times for the entrepreneur-practice owner to contemplate "self-actualization," the peak of Maslow's hierarchy.

"What a man can be, he must be. This need we call self-actualization … It refers to the desire for self-fulfillment, namely, to the tendency for him to become actualized in what he is potentially. This tendency might be phrased as the desire to become more and more what one is, to become everything that one is capable of becoming" (Abraham Maslow).

In the expansion phase, and in consideration of the mature and exit stage, you have the opportunity to take plenty of time to contemplate your future and use your potential. It is too simplistic to say that this is the most important and exciting stage of your career. That would not be true, because the most important stage is the one you are currently in. All previous stages are building blocks for the stage that you are in. It is true to say that the expansion to mature to exit stages are when you can make your greatest contributions to dentistry and to mankind as a whole. You can do this because your time is your own. Day-to-day pressures of your career and family are lessened and you can dedicate yourself to, as the army commercial says, "Be all that you can be." Will you teach? Will you do research? Will you continue to expand your practice? Whatever you decide, if you have pure motivation, you will be successful.

If you decide to expand your practice emotionally, congratulations. Your journey continues. After you have decided how to "self-actualize," you must return to the real world and once again consider your practice in practical terms. You are at a time in your career when you have accumulated much and your aversion to risk should be recalculated from when you originally expanded. This is because when you originally expanded, you had not as much to lose, and a lot more time to recover than now. It is easier to lose something you never really had. The saying "What do I have to lose?" now has an answer. Proceed, because you are driven to, but proceed with a little more caution. You can still walk on the tightrope; just use a net.

There are many ways to expand your practice. The simplest and least risky is to focus on your existing patient base and adapt your practice to their needs. This may include investing in continuing education for the dentists, investing in more modern systems of delivery, and expanding hours, if possible, in existing locations. It may also include review of all marketing strategies and business systems. Keep searching for the future. Stay fresh and current. Never rest on your laurels.

If you plan to expand more externally than internally, you should consider economies of scale. Will expansion result in savings for your practice?

PATIENT BASE

Will expansion expose you to new customers? Will this stress you out too much? (It won't if it helps you be "self-actualized.")

Can you afford to expand? This is when the "tightrope and net" come into play. Previous expansion was a go-for-broke mentality, but this one shouldn't be. You will be able to procure financing at this stage, but should you? I say no. Suze Orman and Dave Ramsey say no, and your Mama and Daddy probably also say no. But if you have good reasons to expand and need debt, go back to Maslow and ask yourself why. (http://www.entrepreneur.com/article/217420)

A very conservative strategy for expansion is to not build more facilities until revenue in the initial locations is three times more revenue than expenses. This is to prepare for the slow revenues in a beginning practice, and the ups and downs in income that happen in all practices but are magnified by more locations.

Although you should be conservative when expanding as opposed to becoming mature, there are good business reasons as well as emotional reasons to expand a late-cycle practice. As the practice and the practitioner-owner move toward the inevitable exit stage, expanding a practice brings greater value to potential buyers. This has great effects on your ability to donate, build your estate for your children, or just increase your ability to build your legacy. Now, isn't that a lot more fun than the stagnating feeling of being mature? You should speed into the exit stage like a Ferrari, not coast in with a clunker.

7

EXIT

"There's a trick to the graceful exit. It begins with the vision to recognize when a job, a life stage, a relationship, is over and to let it go. It means leaving without denying its value."

—ELLEN GOODMAN

L eaving a dental practice, for whatever reason, at whatever age, will always be an emotional decision. Hopefully, you will get to this stage of your career on your own terms.

I advise every practicing dentist I know to skip from expansion to exit, leaving the mature phase out of the picture. Having a mature practice, with dropping production, negative cash flow and profits can drain the soul out of anyone. We cannot control external issues such as illness, death, disability, or other acts of nature that can affect our ability to remain in practice, but we can control how we respond. Expanding resources in a practice is so much better than becoming mature.

Mature practices, typically, have let their facilities decline, their technologies become outmoded, and possibly, their skills lapse. None of these are good for patients and it becomes a downward cycle until the exit stage is the only realistic alternative instead of a life choice. Providing dentistry (or any job), whether individually or as part of a group, should be a passion rather than a chore. At any stage of your career, if you cannot stimulate passion in the act, move to exit. You want to move to the exit stage as a choice rather than have it forced on you. In order to do that, do not become a mature practice.

CHALLENGE

Selling a practice requires a realistic valuation. It may have been years of hard work to build the practice, but what is its real value in the current market place? If you decide to simply close the practice, the challenge is to deal with the financial and psychological aspects of the loss.

FOCUS

Get a proper valuation of your company. Look at your practice operations, management and competitive barriers to make the company worth more to the buyer. Set up legal buy-sell agreements along with a business transition plan.

MONEY SOURCES

Find a business valuation partner. Consult with accountant and financial advisors for the best tax strategy to sell or close a practice.

CHALLENGE OF GETTING A REALISTIC VALUATION

A realistic look at a month in the life of a practice that has *transitioned from the expansion phase directly to the exit phase would look like this:*

WEEK 1

MONDAY

Call from your practice broker telling you he has fielded inquiries from a large corporate group regarding buying your practice. You answer his call from the beach where you spend a portion of each year.

TUESDAY

Friend calls to ask if you can donate toothbrushes to hurricane victims.

WEDNESDAY

Back in the office, you get an update from staff and you get introduced to new staff members.

THURSDAY

Lunch with dean at dental school. He was a dental school classmate of yours.

FRIDAY

Broker calls you again to ask about selling your practice.

WEEK 2

MONDAY

You make appointment with broker and accountant to get your practice evaluated.

TUESDAY

Your youngest child moves out of town today. No chance for local grandchildren.

WEDNESDAY

Charity golf tournament. You have given up golf for many years but are considering getting back into it.

THURSDAY

You spend morning in office visiting with some of your oldest patients. You have not "actually" treated them in years, but they still consider you their dentist, and it is great to see them.

FRIDAY

Your broker and accountant have prepared the practice valuation and now you wait for an offer from the buyer.

WEEK 3

MONDAY

Meeting with lawyer about family trust. If practice sells, what will you do with the proceeds?

TUESDAY

Demo in the office about latest technology "gizmo." How exciting dentistry still is.

WEDNESDAY

Friends at lunch are putting real estate deal together. Not necessarily your thing, but they have been very successful and it might be exciting to try something new.

THURSDAY

Workout with trainer. He says he "is impressed with you" and can't believe your age.

FRIDAY

Offer comes from buyer and it is good. This is going to be a fun weekend.

WEEK 4

MONDAY

ASAP meeting with lawyer, accountant, and practice broker. You discuss a few negotiation points about remaining staff, dental associate compensation, and your personal exit from the practice. You are excited about the future, but this is happening too fast even for an optimist like you.

TUESDAY

Face-to-face meeting with buyers. They respond neutrally to your list of demands and they would like for you to stay on for two years as advisor/consultant. They will pay you a lump sum of 80 percent of value, another 10 percent after year one, and final 10 percent after year two.

WEDNESDAY

After sleeping on it, you will accept the offer. You have discussed this with your wife and you are ready for the next challenge.

THURSDAY

You tell the staff. Hardest thing you have done in your career. They have worked with you forever; they are your family, and although you will still "be around," it won't be the same.

FRIDAY

Lunch with staff.

A realistic look at a month in the life of a practice that has *transitioned from the expansion phase into the mature phase into the exit phase would look like this:*

WEEK 1

MONDAY

Office manager reports to you that Mrs. Jones, who has been a patient for 15 years, is leaving the practice because she cannot miss work at her new job. You have been working 9 a.m. to 4:30 p.m. for 25 years and don't see any reason to change now.

TUESDAY

Fillings all morning. Emergency in the afternoon. Patient needs a root canal and you refer it to the endodontist.

WEDNESDAY

Phone rings all morning, but one receptionist can only answer so many calls. You would add another receptionist, but collections have been slow.

THURSDAY

Mr. Smith, diagnosed with a cracked, nonrestorable tooth last week, and appointed for a bridge today, cancels at the last moment. He has gotten a second opinion because his next-door neighbor got an implant and he wants one too. You have been doing perfectly fine bridges for years and don't see the need for implants.

FRIDAY

You pay bills on Friday mornings and catch up. Your receptionist says you have an emergency patient on the phone, but you tell the patient to call Dr. Jones because, on Fridays, you catch up.

WEEK 2

MONDAY

Sinus headache; no work today. Reschedule. (Why do sinus headaches always come on Monday?)

TUESDAY

Hygienist out sick and you do prophies all afternoon. You tell your wife at dinner you are tired of it all.

WEDNESDAY

The Thompson family calls to tell your office that they have a new PPO insurance and they want to know if you accept it. You never have and you won't start now. They feel bad, but they must change dentists.

THURSDAY

You spend all morning doing fillings on the new pastor's wife's teeth. She is really grateful to you. You feel good, but wish you had more paying patients.

FRIDAY

More bills than money today. No emergencies to bother you. Your wife thinks you need an associate to take the pressure off you.

WEEK 3

MONDAY

You hope your car breaks on the way to work.

TUESDAY

At her recall appointment today, Mrs. Johnson tells you that the gold onlays you did for her 20 years ago feel great. You say you haven't seen her children in a while and she tells you they use the dentist near their work because they have expanded, convenient hours.

WEDNESDAY

Mr. Roberts says he hates his CPAP machine and he wants to know if you can make a snore appliance, like the one his friend at work uses. You tell him you don't do that kind of work, and he says, "That's alright, doc. I will ask my friend for his dentist's card. He is available after hours anyway, so I don't have to miss work."

THURSDAY

You have had it. You make a decision to sell your practice. You have that cabin in the woods you want to spend more time at.

FRIDAY

You sit down with your last five years of tax returns and decide what you think your practice is worth.

WEEK 4

MONDAY

You are happy to drive to work for the first day that you can remember. You have a lunch appointment with a broker to list the practice.

TUESDAY

Broker spends afternoon in office. Girls wonder what is going on.

WEDNESDAY

Meet with broker after work. His appraisal is way less than what you had expected! You have worked your whole life for this! He says declining production every year, declining area, older equipment, and a deteriorating facility all make it less attractive to buyers than you had thought.

THURSDAY

You spend the day thinking about how you can update, but you really don't want to spend the money and you don't have the motivation any more.

FRIDAY

You call the broker and list the practice at his price. You somehow feel relieved because you will get to spend more time at the cabin.

Wow! Those are two different tunes. Obviously, they are exaggerations of two very different stories. I have seen both stories many times and I think you know which one I like telling the best.

Remember, all life-cycle stages are building blocks for the next phase. One dentist reached a certain level of establishment and never wanted to leave. The other dentist moved into the expansion stage and never left. Also, remember that expansion does not only mean building a monetary monster. Expansion also means growth and stimulation of dental skills, training of staff, and all methods that keep every day fresh. When things quit being fun and exciting, do something different. If you do that, you will always be in expansion.

We have discussed the conditions possible when one reaches the exit stage. Let's address actually exiting.

Focus on proper valuations, practice operations, and competitive barriers. Whether you are approached to sell your practice, or list the practice yourself, you will want to get a realistic valuation of your practice. An accountant, business broker, or specialized valuation expert can be helpful in appraising your practice.

Unfortunately, there is no standardized universally accepted formula that an evaluator may use to establish the value of a dental practice. There are many objective factors that should be considered to determine the value. There are also many subjective factors unique to dentistry that are just as important. Although there are many methods that may be used to value a dental practice, most approaches tend to fall into these three methods:

ASSET-BASED VALUATION

The asset based valuation method calculates the value of the dental practice that may be sold. These assets may be valued based on the original cost, the book value (reduced by depreciation) or the replacement value or appraised value. The shortcoming of evaluating a practice based solely on its assets is that the practice's earnings and cash flow are not considered. Additionally, it is very difficult to accurately appraise the value of the goodwill of a practice. Any valuation of a business in the services industry should include an analysis of the profitability of the venture. As a result, the asset-based method is rarely used without consulting one of the following two methods:

MARKET COMPARISON VALUATION

The market comparison valuation method identifies similar practices that have been sold and applies certain ratios of those recent practice sales to the practice being sold. Several different valuation ratios are used, including the ratio of the sales price to discretionary cash flow, sales price to annual net profits, or sales price to annual revenues of the practice. Viewing recent sales would seem a good indicator of practice value, but it often ignores the unique nature of a given practice.

INCOME-BASED VALUATION

The income-based valuation method identifies the projected future cash flow of the practice. The amount of cash flow is then capitalized, discounted, or multiplied, based on one of the following methods:

1. the present value of future earnings

2. a capitalization of excess earnings valuation

3. a multiple of discretionary earnings valuation

A simple way to get a thumbnail idea of what your practice is worth today is to divide last year's collections by two and add the value of all the furniture, dental equipment, supplies, and computers (complete contents). Find a broker you are comfortable with. Ask for referrals, as often the brokers are more interested in their commission than they are in you. Your broker will ask you for recent income statements, equipment valuations, production collection reports, accounts receivable aging report, relationship with insurance PPOs, tax returns, and on and on. Have these prepared and ready to go. The buyer or bankers financing the sale for the buyer will have tons more questions, so be patient.

Once the practice is listed, hopefully, you will be deluged with calls. You will want to be discreet with patients and staff, because you don't want everybody jumping off the ship.

Follow this checklist prepared by my friend Dan Lewis, the best practice broker in America.

SELLER'S PRACTICE SALE CHECK LIST

---

1. CONDUCT STAFF MEETING(S) TO INFORM OF TRANSITION:

❑ Discuss reason for transition. Inform staff of use of transition consultant.

❑ Discuss time line and expectations.

❑ Discuss need for "status quo" in practice operation.

❑ Emphasize need for *team effort* in achieving success for all.

❑ Emphasize need for confidentiality (other dentists and their staff).

❑ Express hope that all staff will stay; give purchaser a chance.

❑ Discuss needs of office to prepare for sale: cleanup, painting, repairs.

❑ Discuss possible scripting to handle patient inquiries.

2. CONTACT PROFESSIONAL ADVISORS

❑ Attorney:

    ❑ Do initial planning on sale impact.

❑ Accountant:

❑ Understand tax implications of sale.

❑ Discuss timing of sale.

❑ Bank:

    ❑ Discuss debts to be paid from sales proceeds.

    ❑ Be aware of prepayment penalties or obstacles.

❑ Landlord:

    ❑ Discuss need to notify landlord and understand options available for transfer/assignment.

❑ Others:

    ❑ financial planners

    ❑ consultant insurance agent

3. SELLER AND PURCHASER CONFERENCES

❑ Discuss employee's salaries, benefits, bonuses.

❑ Discuss sick day and vacation policies.

❑ Provide/obtain employees' salary histories and work records.

❑ Review fee schedule with purchaser.

❑ Discuss historical policies for warranty work.

❑ Discuss office/personal policies for pro bono or discounted work.

❑ Discuss office policy manual.

❑ Review new patient procedures.

❑ Review case presentation procedures.

- ❏ Review minimum of 10 active patient charts for diagnosis compatibility.

- ❏ Discuss current suppliers and labs.

- ❏ Discuss specialists used.

- ❏ Discuss office staff meeting policies/frequencies.

- ❏ Review list of patient charts to be kept (family, friends).

- ❏ Review ongoing treatments of special needs patients.

4. PRIOR TO CLOSING

- ❏ Prepare letters of introduction:
    - ❏ patient letter;
    - ❏ referral sources;
    - ❏ other professionals;
    - ❏ send out concurrently with closing—not before closing;
    - ❏ seller normally composes and purchaser revises and approves.

- ❏ Notify current lien holders of impending sale:
    - ❏ Obtain payoff amounts.

- ❏ Investigate need for personal health insurance carrier change.

- ❏ Contact landlord to complete lease assignment to purchaser:
    - ❏ Prepare office lease if seller is landlord.

- ❏ Arrange for transfer of software license(s) dental software:
    - ❏ business software

- ❑ imaging software and hardware

❑ Arrange for transfer of maintenance agreements:

- ❑ computer hardware and software

- ❑ postage meter

- ❑ copy machine

- ❑ security system

❑ Arrange for transfer of credit card servicing account.

❑ Request transfer of service agreement form from telephone company.

❑ Run accounts receivable report for planning and write off uncollectable accounts.

❑ Check status of patient credit balances.

5. CONCURRENT WITH CLOSING

❑ Run final accounts receivable and credit balance report.

❑ Back up all practice data to the date of closing and archive.

❑ Notify service providers of termination of accounts:

- ❑ oxygen and nitrous tanks

- ❑ waste disposal

- ❑ long-distance carrier

- ❑ dental supply companies

- ❑ office supplies laboratories

❑ direct vendors

❑ display advertising vendors

❑ Notify state board of practice sale.

❑ Notify state employment/workforce commission of practice sale.

❑ Notify local office of radiological health/control for X-ray ownership change.

❑ Notify state secretary of state regarding status of change of business location (within your state) or termination of business.

❑ Notify the following of address change and/or retirement from local dental society:

❑ American Dental Association

❑ state dental association

❑ other professional societies

❑ malpractice insurance carrier

❑ magazine subscriptions

❑ bank and credit card companies

❑ other suppliers

❑ professional journals

❑ Schedule transfer of utilities:

❑ electric provider

❑ gas company

❑ city services: water and waste

❑ Complete telephone company phone transfer:

    ❑ Obtain transfer of service agreement.

❑ Coordinate transfer of practice health insurance plan.

❑ Notify county taxing authority of business ownership change.

EPILOGUE

I have tried to paint a realistic picture of each stage of the dental practice lifecycle. I also hope to have provided some insight into clues with dealing with a dental career. I will leave you with a few caveats:

1. I have given some references to time frames, when certain practice cycle events could happen in real life. The dental practice life cycles can be accelerated simply by mastering the stage you are in and importing some of the techniques from the stage immediately following the stage you are in. For example, in any phase, if you want to move forward faster, consider marketing with Chrisad (www.chrisad.com) and practice management with Breakaway (www.breakawaypracticeseminars.com), or Stratus dental (www.stratusdental.com).

2. The purpose of this book is not to be judgmental of anyone's career choices or methods of practice. It is, hopefully, a way for you to understand that anything is possible. Life and your career are yours to enjoy, and you should not limit your horizons. Opportunities in dentistry are endless. Computer scientist Alan Kay said, "The best way to predict the future is to invent it." The best way to build a fantastic career in dentistry is to dream it.

3. There have been many people who have influenced me personally and professionally throughout my career. If you want to be successful, do what successful people do.

4. Be happy to share great ideas with your colleagues; don't horde them. Besides helping someone else, you never know what good will come back to you.

5. Always enjoy the journey. Although we always point to the end goal, first, you will never get there, and second, you will get there soon enough.

MUSINGS FROM THE AUTHOR DURING THE WRITING OF THIS BOOK

In September 2011 I was asked to speak at a dental marketing meeting in Boston as an "after picture" to discuss what Chrisad marketing had done for our practice. I had been working with Chrisad for about eight years and our original office had grown 150 percent. We had also added another practice that grew fivefold. I was very honored to be asked to speak. Members of my staff, who were in attendance, told me they were shocked that I could speak in front of a large group. I told them that I felt comfortable because I was simply telling a true story. Also, after practicing dentistry for 30 years, I felt I had many stories to tell. A book seemed like a good outlet for me. I contacted my publisher and designed an outline for this book. In August 2012, with great excitement, I began writing and corresponding with my editor. This is an instructional manual on how I have managed a dental career. I thought I was an expert. The jury is still out.

It is important for dentists at any level of their career to seek answers to practice management as well technical advancements.

In July 2012 I was referred to "Breakaway," a course by Dr. Scott Leune that helps organize and run dental practices, including group practices. We took our front office staff. We found the course exciting because Dr. Leune suggested many of the methods we had already employed in our offices. What we learned is that he had organized and documented his methods much better than we had and we took his training manuals home with the purpose of creating manuals for our staff that would describe not only job duties but also how to perform them. We saw this as a major step in our attempt to stream-line. However, it became very time consuming and difficult for us to put together. Although hard for us to perform in practice, I was impressed with the manuals given to us by Breakaway and decided the next step for our practice development and me was to write a book to be used as our manual and as a guide for our practices.

Like everyone nowadays, when I have a question I turn to Google. I Googled how to write a book in August 2012 and found Advantage Media Group. They set me up with an editor. While sitting in a golf cart with my friends on the practice tee, I made an outline with my editor. We arranged for phone "interviews" to flesh out topics from our outline. I would call her on Saturday morning from wherever I was. I was traveling a lot at that time. The weekly phone calls and their different locations began to have an effect on my thinking process. The prep for the call during the week made me really evaluate why and how we managed our practices. The preparation and research would also take me into other practice methods and I began to realize that although I had a lot of knowledge, I needed to study more. The phone calls from different locales (the Texas A&M Florida Gator tailgate in College Station Texas, a New York City hotel room, a DC park near the White House) reconfirmed what a great career and job choice we have made. Being out of the office is good for thinking and planning. I think the lesson learned in stepping away from the office is not only a great idea but also imperative for planning. I like to make important decisions about work, or life in general, away from the office. Write things down for permanent introspection. (Write your own book. You will think more about your actions because print holds you accountable.) Understand that business, like everything else, is a process, and although I can write down great words of wisdom to help on your road, it is always a journey, and I have not reached the destination yet and don't really expect to.

Nothing ever stays the same. Man plans and the Lord laughs. In September 2012 my daughter got engaged. My wife and I were thrilled. We flew to DC for the surprise engagement. In October, on the way to the airport for a trip to Germany, a broker called and asked if I was interested in selling our satellite practice. Although it had not been for sale, I had been become restless, and was looking for a change. The practice had been appraised six months previously, and I agreed to sell. It was a great deal for me. But now I had a whole new job. The transition involved contracts, tax planning, accountants and lawyers while the day-to-day practice continued. Dentists and practice managers need to be adaptable to all opportunities, threats and our changing environment. We also need to stay current with the general business world. Keeping our head solely in dental journals may make us better practitioners, but in order to maintain a viable practice where we have a place to provide beautiful dentistry, we must stay aware of the dental and general business world outside. I started studying to become accredited by the Association of Accredited Small Business Consultants (www.aasbc.com). It gives me more knowledge of accounting principles, balance sheets, profit and loss statements, fraud protection, general marketing, and basic business language. This comes in handy when speaking to bankers, brokers and accountants. I have been a dentist for 30 years and have studied all disciplines of dentistry, which, although necessary for quality care are not more important to being a successful dentist, in today's environment, than business skills.

Shortly after selling our satellite practice in December 2012, another broker called and said a very similar rural practice had come onto the market. We drove to the country, visited the practice and found it attractive because it had the same demographics as the practice we had just sold. We had owned our satellite practice for nine years, and grown it from two chairs and three employees in a broken-down, prefabricated building, to eight chairs in a modern 3500-square-foot building. The new practice also had two chairs and two employees. Because it was in an area with a lot of potential, we bought it—lawyers, accountants and brokers again.

While doing my usual surfing for Internet answers, I came across a practice management course called Stratus dental www.stratusdental.com. Managing more than one office, staff training, communication, scheduling efficiency, overhead efficiency, supply cost, fighting the big chains were all big issues to our practices. Stratus addressed these issues through literature and phone conversations. I traveled to Oakland, California, for a one-day Stratus informational meeting and found it fascinating. Through online and phone conversations, management and training systems are set up for all our offices, and conceivably, many more. We signed up with Stratus in July and a whirlwind of activity has occurred. Our computer software has been linked to their computers to give me daily office financial updates. Our telephones are monitored to evaluate phone answering efficiency—namely, calls answered and missed, and where referrals are coming from for marketing ROI analysis. The best part is that training for every team member is available for all the things we need to work on. I am more excited for the future than I have been in 10 years.

During the course of my 30-year practice life cycle, I have seen dentistry change in many aspects. In 1982 most treatment was being delivered in solo practitioner offices. Typically, one hygienist performed prophies and one or, possibly, two assistants worked with the dentist. Most practices offered 9–5 schedules (or "banking hours") and were closed on Wednesday or Friday afternoons. A 4–6 chair practice was considered large. The dentist's goal was to keep himself busy all the time. Most practices did not accept payment via dental insurance. It was often considered a breach of professionalism to accept insurance as payment. An elitism existed in the profession, especially among the older, more established dentists, who were raised in an era when dentists could put their name on a sign and patients would pour in. It was definitely a seller's market then.

Because solo dentists were as "busy" as they wanted to be, income was more influenced by fee increases, or by higher fees for more complex cases and, later, by improvements in technology or inner office efficiency to provide more services at a faster rate or more cost-effective manner.

Schedules were organized more for the convenience of the staff and dentist than the patient. Reception areas were, typically, quiet, sometimes lit only by table lamps and separated from the receptionist's work area by a frosted-glass window. Patients would ring a bell to announce their arrival, and a grumpy receptionist would tell them, "Please be seated, and the doctor will be right with you." This would mean that the doctor would be with you when he got around to it. The patient would dutifully have a seat and wait as patiently as possible, reading old *National Geographic* magazines until an assistant dressed like a nurse would open the door to the treatment area and ask the patient to go with her. The patient would follow the assistant down the hallway, where she would open the door to the operatory. The patient would have a seat and the assistant would leave and shut the door.

The patient would bide his time looking at scary instruments neatly laid out in front of him while indelibly imprinting on his memory the aroma of zinc oxide and eugenol (the smell of a dental office). Maybe he would study the nautical map on the wall. But mostly, the patient would sit petrified, alone in the small room, waiting for the door to open and a man in a barber gown to enter.

In the late sixties, many dentists still had belt-driven hand pieces and many still stood as they treated the patient. By 1982 most dentists sat and belt-driven hand pieces were for the real old-timers.

If anesthesia was indicated, the dentist would administer the injection and leave the room, shutting the door behind him. The patient would sit alone and the Bill Cosby skit would come to life.

The fancy delivery unit of the day was an Executive by Pelton Crane. If you had an Executive, you were cool! It was like driving a Porsche.

Believe it or not, until 1982 people could smoke in the dental office, and sometimes even the dentist would smoke in the operatory. Ask your mom. People could smoke everywhere, even in doctors' and dentists' offices.

Composite fillings were used only in the front of the mouth, and shades were limited. Silver fillings were the most common treatment for the back of the mouth. Gold foil was considered an excellent restoration. Silver points were considered acceptable root canal fillers. Porcelain laminates were being promoted by progressive "cosmetic dentists" who would not accept the common notion that being able to differentiate real teeth from fillings was not such a bad thing, and it was okay to try to make people's teeth look better even if nothing was physically wrong with them. This concept changed the way dentists and patients perceived our profession. We offered a service that was optional and not a necessity. And we wanted people to know what was possible. So, many progressive dentists started to advertise. This really caused a schism, as the old school traditionalists were appalled by advertising and what was happening to our profession.

Cosmetic treatment, and advertising were not the only external forces changing dentistry in the '80s. Delta Dental is the largest dental plan system in the United States. Delta Dental was originated in 1954 with the formation of dental services in California, Oregon and Washington. Dental insurance plans were sprouting in the 1970s.

Dental insurance companies, in the interest of staying competitive, developed networks, PPOs, and HMOs, whereby dentists would contract with the insurance companies to provide either lower fees or even "capitation" plans to offer lower-cost dentistry to patients. It sounded great to patients, but it was the beginning of the end of the solo dentist with his name on the sign and patients pouring in.

Old, established practices were able to maintain the old paradigm, but younger dentists, in the name of paying bills, succumbed to the pressure of the insurance companies. Not only did dentists routinely accept insurance assignment as payment, many signed on as "preferred providers" who would be part of a network of doctors, providing fees at the lower rates. These PPO dentists were often scorned or shunned at meetings and conventions and were often assumed to be inferior in the care they provided. How could quality care be performed at such low fees?

Insurance, cosmetic dentistry, and advertising—a revolution was on. Many dentists did, in fact, perform inferior treatment, rationalizing the fact that patients drawn to their practices by advertisements of low fees did not deserve excellent care. Many dentists, however, still loving their profession and their patients, and taking their oath to provide the best possible care seriously, began to develop systems that would provide efficient, cost-saving mechanisms for a highly successful practice with a high quality of care. The paradigm had shifted.

When external forces began to have as much influence on the dental practice as the dentist himself, many dentists struggled with the new demands of running a practice. It was no longer enough to be an excellent practitioner to be successful. The new dental practice had to have an excellent manager as well. Some dentists resisted and withered. Some became very adept at running not only a practice but also a business. Some compromised by hiring management consultants to help.

Of course, with the expansion of size, scope and productivity of dental "businesses," the real corporate world wanted to get involved, and in the '80s, large corporations and venture capitalists saw an opportunity. Now we can never turn back. I still went to meetings in 2013 at which old-timers scoffed at the notion of expanded duty assistants, advertising and corporate dentistry. I laugh at their indignation because burying one's head in the sand won't make contemporary practices go away. Often, excellent dentistry is being performed in corporate dental "clinics" and to ignore it and deny it won't change it. Fortunately, these old-timers won't have to worry about it for long because they are at the end of their careers.

Recognition of the real facts and the ability to adapt properly is the key to success. Fortune favors the bold.

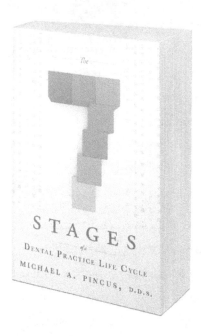

How can you use this book?

MOTIVATE

EDUCATE

THANK

INSPIRE

PROMOTE

CONNECT

Why have a custom version of
The Seven Stages of a Dental Practice Life Cycle?

- Build personal bonds with customers, prospects, employees, donors, and key constituencies

- Develop a long-lasting reminder of your event, milestone, or celebration

- Provide a keepsake that inspires change in behavior and change in lives

- Deliver the ultimate "thank you" gift that remains on coffee tables and bookshelves

- Generate the "wow" factor

Books are thoughtful gifts that provide a genuine sentiment that other promotional items cannot express. They promote employee discussions and interaction, reinforce an event's meaning or location, and they make a lasting impression. Use your book to say "Thank You" and show people that you care.

The Seven Stages of a Dental Practice Life Cycle is available in bulk quantities and in customized versions at special discounts for corporate, institutional, and educational purposes. To learn more please contact our Special Sales team at:

1.866.775.1696 • sales@advantageww.com • www.AdvantageSpecialSales.com

Printed in the USA
CPSIA information can be obtained
at www.ICGtesting.com
JSHW012040140824
68134JS00033B/3175

9 781599 323701